Asthma

Editors

CATHERINE D. CATRAMBONE
LINDA M. FOLLENWEIDER

NURSING CLINICS
OF NORTH AMERICA

www.nursing.theclinics.com

Consulting Editor
STEPHEN D. KRAU

March 2013 • Volume 48 • Number 1

ELSEVIER

1600 John F. Kennedy Boulevard • Suite 1800 • Philadelphia, Pennsylvania, 19103-2899

http://www.theclinics.com

NURSING CLINICS OF NORTH AMERICA Volume 48, Number 1
March 2013 ISSN 0029-6465, ISBN-13: 978-1-4557-7125-7

Editor: Katie Saunders
Developmental Editor: Donald Mumford

Nursing Clinics of North America (ISSN 0029-6465) is published quarterly by Elsevier Inc., 360 Park Avenue South, New York, NY 10010-1710. Months of issue are March, June, September, and December. Periodicals postage paid at New York, NY and additional mailing offices. Subscription price per year is, $144.00 (US individuals), $374.00 (US institutions), $260.00 (international individuals), $456.00 (international institutions), $210.00 (Canadian individuals), $456.00 (Canadian institutions), $79.00 (US students), and $129.00 (international students). To receive student/resident rate, orders must be accompanied by name of affiliated institution, date of term, and the signature of program/residency coordinator on institution letterhead. Orders will be billed at individual rate until proof of status is received. Foreign air speed delivery is included in all *Clinics* subscription prices. All prices are subject to change without notice. **POSTMASTER:** Send address changes to *Nursing Clinics*, Elsevier Health Sciences Division, Subscription Customer Service, 3251 Riverport Lane, Maryland Heights, MO 63043. **Customer Service: Telephone: 1-800-654-2452** (U.S. and Canada); **1-314-447-8871 (outside U.S. and Canada). Fax: 1-314-447-8029. E-mail: journalscustomerservice-usa@elsevier.com** (for print support) and **journalsonlinesupport-usa@elsevier.com** (for online support).

Nursing Clinics of North America is covered in *EMBASE/Excerpta Medica, MEDLINE/PubMed (Index Medicus), Social Sciences Citation Index, Current Contents, ASCA, Cumulative Index to Nursing, RNdex Top 100,* and Allied Health Literature and International Nursing Index (INI).

Printed and bound by CPI Group (UK) Ltd, Croydon, CR0 4YY
Transferred to Digital Printing, 2013

Contributors

CONSULTING EDITOR

STEPHEN D. KRAU, PhD, RN, CNE
Associate Professor, Vanderbilt University School of Nursing, South Nashville, Tennessee

EDITORS

CATHERINE D. CATRAMBONE, PhD, RN, FAAN
Associate Professor, Adult Health and Gerontological Nursing, Rush University College of Nursing, Chicago, Illinois

LINDA M. FOLLENWEIDER, MS, APN, C-FNP
Senior Consultant, Health Management Associates, Chicago, Illinois

AUTHORS

ELLEN A. BECKER, PhD, RRT-NPS, RPFT, AE-C, FAARC
Associate Professor, Department of Respiratory Care, Rush University College of Health Professions, Chicago, Illinois

ANNA L. EDWARDS, NP-C, MSN
Glendora, CA

RAECHEL FERRY-ROONEY, MSN, APRN-ANP
Instructor, Adult and Gerontology Nurse Practitioner Program, Clinical Faculty at College of Nursing, Rush University; Adult Nurse Practitioner, University of Illinois Medical Center, Chicago, Illinois

LINDA M. FOLLENWEIDER, MS, CNP
Health Management Associates, Chicago, Illinois

MAUREEN GEORGE, PhD, RN, AE-C, FAAN
Assistant Professor, Department of Family and Community Health, University of Pennsylvania School of Nursing; Senior Fellow, Center for Health Behavior Research, University of Pennsylvania, Philadelphia, Pennsylvania

CATHERINE "CASEY" S. JONES, PhD, RN, ANP-C, AE-C
Texas Pulmonary and Critical Care Consultants, PA, Texas Woman's University, Bedford, Texas

KATHRYN KILLEEN, MSN, APN, ACNP-BC, CCNS
Advanced Practice Nurse, Division of Pulmonary and Critical Care Medicine, Department of Adult Critical Care Nursing, Rush University Medical Center, Chicago, Illinois

ANISSA LAMBERTINO, MPH
Health Management Associates, Chicago, Illinois

LAURA LEMMENES, MS/MBA, APN, DNP
Family Nurse Practitioner, Advocate Health Care, Chicago, Illinois

AMY B. MANION, PhD, RN, PNP
Pediatric Nurse Practitioner, Northwestern Children's Practice; Assistant Professor, College of Nursing, Rush University, Chicago, Illinois

MOLLY A. MARTIN, MD, MAPP
Assistant Professor, Department of Preventive Medicine, Rush University Medical Center, Chicago, Illinois

KAREN L. MEYERSON, MSN, RN, FNP-C, AE-C
Manager, Asthma Network of West Michigan, Grand Rapids, Michigan

ELIZABETH SKORA, MSN, APN, ANP-BC
Clinical Faculty, Instructor, Department of Adult and Gerontological Nursing, Rush University College of Nursing, Chicago, Illinois

MAXIM TOPAZ, RN, MA
Fulbright Fellow, University of Haifa, Israel; PhD Student, University of Pennsylvania School of Nursing, Philadelphia, Pennsylvania

LINDA SUE VAN ROEYEN, MS, CSN, CCRP, FNP-BC
Ann and Robert H. Lurie Children's Hospital of Chicago; Pulmonary Habilitation Program, Adjunct Faculty, DePaul University, Chicago, Illinois

Contents

Incidence and prevalence rates of asthma can vary greatly according to population and location. The National Heart and Blood Institute of the National Institutes of Health defines asthma as a common chronic disorder of the airways that involves a complex interaction of airflow obstruction, bronchial hyperresponsiveness, and an underlying inflammation. This article uses the most common definitions and diagnostic methods for asthma. In 2009 there were 2.1 million asthma-related emergency department (ED) visits. ED visits lend an opportunity for providers to identify and intervene in the care of patients whose asthma is poorly controlled.

Asthma is a chronic inflammatory disorder that is characterized by 3 distinct responses in the airways: inflammation, hyperresponsiveness, and remodeling. Clinical diagnosis of asthma is often based on the presence of symptoms, such as cough, wheeze, breathlessness, and chest tightness; but the presence of these symptoms is not exclusive to asthma, and clinical correlation with spirometry and other diagnostic testing is essential. Once a diagnosis of asthma is established, the focus of care should be toward control of the disease. This article discusses the pathophysiology, diagnosis, and clinical assessment of asthma in the adult patient population.

Asthma remains a significant public health burden in the United States. Primary care providers are in an ideal position to be able to target treatment for their patients on an individual basis. It is important to determine the level of control and then base treatment on both the severity and activity of disease and the ability of the patient to be adherent to the therapy regimen. Because prescription medications along with office visits represent most asthma expenses, it is imperative to choose wisely from among the quick-relief and the long-term control medications to find the right choice for your patient.

of IgE-mediated sensitization and bronchial hyperresponsiveness occurs with OA. Also, extreme short-term chemical exposures versus a cumulative effect of chemical exposures will need continued evaluation to determine tolerable levels that do not cause harm. Health care providers often seek guidance from NIOSH, which sponsors ongoing research and training related to workplace exposures.

The incidence of pediatric asthma in the United States creates a huge financial burden to the economy as well as a negative impact on child health. Identification and elimination of asthma triggers are helpful in reducing asthma exacerbations. The incidence of asthma is higher in African American and underserved populations. Improved management of pediatric asthma leads to improved school performance, improved mental health, and general well-being.

Asthma remains a serious health risk in the United States, particularly among children from low-income families. This article presents an overview of the Asthma Network of West Michigan, the local asthma coalition serving West Michigan, and its intensive home-based case management model for individuals with uncontrolled asthma. The Asthma Network is believed to be the first grassroots asthma coalition in the nation to contract with health plans and obtain reimbursement for these services. The Asthma Network's program has had a positive impact on health care use as well as cost savings, and its model has been replicated in other communities.

NURSING CLINICS
OF NORTH AMERICA

DOWNLOAD
Free App!

Review Articles
THE CLINICS

NOW AVAILABLE FOR YOUR iPhone and iPad

Preface

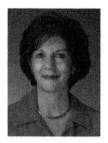 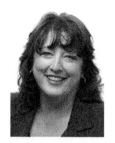

Catherine D. Catrambone, PhD, RN, FAAN   Linda M. Follenweider, MS, APN, C-FNP
Editors

Asthma is a chronic disease that affects adults and children. Asthma impacts health systems, health providers, and individual health, clinically and economically. The burden of asthma remains a significant public health concern nationally and globally. In a 2012 report, the Centers for Disease Control and Prevention reported that the number of persons with asthma has risen steadily over the past decade from 20.3 to 25.7 million in the United States.[1] In 2007, The National Asthma Education and Prevention Program of the National Heart, Lung, and Blood Institute published the most recent Expert Panel Report 3: *Guidelines for the Diagnosis and Management of Asthma* that provides a comprehensive approach to the diagnosis and management of asthma.[2] Despite the availability of published asthma guidelines for over 2 decades, widespread adherence to guideline-recommended care remains a goal yet to be achieved.[3–6] This issue of *Nursing Clinics of North America* provides a broad range of asthma-related topics including the state of asthma in the United States, overview of guideline-recommended asthma care, selected developments in asthma research, asthma management in various settings, and an innovative state-level asthma program.

The issue begins with an overview from Follenweider and Lambertino of the epidemiology of asthma and addresses national and global prevalence, morbidity and mortality, indoor and outdoor environmental risk factors, and emotional factors related to asthma.

The next 4 articles provide a framework for the diagnosis and care of asthma. Killeen and Skora discuss the pathophysiology, diagnosis, and clinical assessment of the adult client with asthma. Ferry-Rooney and Damitz, through a case-presentation, discuss goals and pharmacologic treatment of asthma. Similarly, Jones, Becker, Catrambone, and Martin discuss a guideline-approach to asthma management with an emphasis on severity and control and considerations for improving guideline adherence. Given the current economic climate within health care and incentive structures, Edward's article addresses the importance of asthma action plans and self-management and their impact on key outcome variables stressing health literacy and its impact on asthma management.

Current asthma research is featured in the following 2 articles. Topaz and George present a comprehensive, systematic review of complementary and alternative medicine (CAM) for asthma self-management. The authors address the body of research on CAM use for asthma in both children and adults and the safety and effectiveness of

---

Nurs Clin N Am 48 (2013) ix–x
http://dx.doi.org/10.1016/j.cnur.2013.01.002
0029-6465/13/$ – see front matter © 2013 Published by Elsevier Inc.   **nursing.theclinics.com**

these treatments. The article by Manion features an overview of the research related to asthma and obesity with an emphasis on dose-effect and implications for management of asthma.

The final 3 articles focus on asthma management in the workplace, school, and community. Lemmenes defines work-related asthma (WRA) and provides a detailed discussion of the major divisions of WRA including work-exacerbated asthma and occupational asthma, including sensitizer-induced and irritant-induced asthma. This author addresses pathophysiology, testing, and measures to eliminate or control workplace exposure. In this pediatric-focused article, Van Royen discusses asthma in the home, including the identification of and methods for eliminating asthma triggers. In the school setting, she reviews the impact of asthma—related absenteeism and discusses the role of school-based health centers, legislation, education programs, and health provider care in the school setting. In the article by Meyerson, the elements, impact, and expansion of an innovative model of home-based case management for asthma in Michigan are described.

Catherine D. Catrambone, PhD, RN, FAAN
Associate Professor, Adult Health and Gerontological Nursing
Rush University College of Nursing
600 S. Paulina, 1064B Armour Academic Center
Chicago, IL 60612, USA

Linda M. Follenweider, MS, APN, C-FNP
Senior Consultant, Health Management Associates
180 North LaSalle, Suite 2305
Chicago, IL 60601, USA

E-mail addresses:
cathy_catrambone@rush.edu (C.D. Catrambone)
lfollenweider@healthmanagement.com (L.M. Follenweider)

REFERENCES

1. Moorman JE, Akinbami LJ, Bailey CM, et al. National Surveillance of Asthma: United States, 2001–2010. National Center for Health Statistics. Vital Health Stat 2012;3(35):3.
2. National Institutes of Health National Heart Blood and Lung Institute. Guidelines for the diagnosis and management of asthma (EPR-3). Full report 2007. National Institutes of Health National Heart Blood and Lung Institute; 2007 NIH Publication 08-5846. Available at: http://www.nhlbi.nih.gov/guidelines/asthma/asthgdln.htm. Accessed February 1, 2013.
3. Navaratnam P. Physician adherence to the national asthma prescribing guidelines: evidence from national outpatient survey data in the United States. AnnAllergy Asthma Immunol 2008;100(3):216.
4. Rance K, O'Laughlen M, Ting S. Improving asthma care for African American children by increasing national asthma guideline adherence. J Pediatr Health Care 2011;25(4):235–49.
5. Weinstein A. The potential of asthma adherence management to enhance asthma guidelines. Ann Allergy Asthma Immunol 2011;106(4):283–91.
6. Wisnivesky J, Lorenzo J, Lyn Cook R, et al. Barriers to adherence to asthma management guidelines among inner-city primary care providers. Ann Allergy Asthma Immunol 2008;101(3):264–70.

Erratum

Refers to: "A Report on a National Study of Doctoral Nursing Faculty" and Contributors list

By H. Michael Dreher, Mary Ellen Smith Glasgow, Frances H. Cornelius, Anand Bhattacharya

December 2012 Volume 47 Issue 4

ISSN 0029-6465

In the December 2012 issue of Nursing Clinics of North America, an error was made in the article, "A Report on a National Study of Doctoral Nursing Faculty" and the Contributors page. Dr H. Michael Dreher's affiliation information was incorrectly listed. His correct credentials and title are: H. Michael Dreher, PhD, RN, FAAN, Associate Professor of the Department of Advanced Nursing Roles at the College of Nursing & Health Professions of Drexel University.

We apologize for this oversight.

http://dx.doi.org/10.1016/j.cnur.2013.01.001

Erratum

Epidemiology of Asthma in the United States

Linda M. Follenweider, MS, CNP*, Anissa Lambertino, MPH

KEYWORDS

• Asthma • Epidemiology • Incidence • Diagnosis

KEY POINTS

• Accurate data on the prevalence and incidence of asthma to inform research and clinical practice has been hindered by the lack of a consistent method of identifying and diagnosing asthma, both clinically and in studies of asthma.
• The National Heart and Blood Institute of the National Institutes of Health defines asthma as a common chronic disorder of the airways that involves a complex interaction of airflow obstruction, bronchial hyperresponsiveness, and an underlying inflammation.
• In 2009 there were 2.1 million asthma-related emergency department (ED) visits. ED visits provide an opportunity for providers to identify and intervene in the care of patients whose asthma is poorly controlled.
• Other factors that can exacerbate asthma symptoms include indoor allergens such as pet dander, outdoor environmental irritants such as exhaust, and emotional factors such as violence in the home.

EPIDEMIOLOGY OF ASTHMA

Accurate data on the prevalence and incidence of asthma to inform research and clinical practice has been hindered by the lack of a consistent method of identifying and diagnosing asthma, both clinically and in studies of asthma. Studies that differ in the definition and diagnosis of asthma create difficulty in comparisons. This article uses the most common definitions and diagnostic methods for asthma. The National Heart and Blood Institute of the National Institutes of Health defines asthma as a common chronic disorder of the airways that involves a complex interaction of airflow obstruction, bronchial hyperresponsiveness, and an underlying inflammation. This interaction can be highly variable among patients and within patients over time.[1] Asthma is a disease that affects adults and children and occurs in all populations and locations across the globe. Incidence and prevalence rates can vary greatly according to population and location.

Health Management Associates, 180 N. LaSalle Street, Chicago, IL 60601, USA
* Corresponding author.
E-mail address: follenweider@gmail.com

GLOBAL IMPACT OF ASTHMA

In 2004, the Global Initiative for Asthma (GINA) combined data from the International Study of Asthma and Allergies (ISAAC) study and the European Community Respiratory Health Survey (ECRHS) to provide global estimates on the burden of asthma. These data were collected between 1992 and 1996 and 1988 and 1994, respectively. The GINA report estimated an asthma prevalence rate for countries that ranged from the lowest prevalence in Macau (0.7%) to the highest prevalence in Scotland (18.4%). The analysis was limited because of the different surveys and sampling methodologies used by the 2 studies as well as different definitions of asthma and age groups.[2] The World Health Organization (WHO) designed the World Health Survey (WHS), which allowed for the standardization of data collected between 2002 and 2003 across the world in 6 continents and a broad range of countries, which allows for within-country and between-country comparisons. In an analysis of the WHS data concerning asthma that was performed by To and colleagues[2] in 2012, the global prevalence of doctor-diagnosed asthma in adults was estimated at 4.3% and the prevalence of clinical asthma (asthma diagnosed through less stringent methods) was 4.5%, with a range of 1% in Vietnam and 21.5% in Australia. Definition for clinical asthma was based on doctor-diagnosed asthma and/or a positive response to either of 2 questions: "Have you ever been treated for asthma?" or "Have you been taking any medications or treatment for asthma during the last 2 weeks?" The 5 countries with the highest burden of asthma were Australia (21.1%), Sweden (20.2%), United Kingdom (18.2%), the Netherlands (15.3%), and Brazil (13.0%). In addition, the WHS looked at clinical and behavioral data on the participants. Almost a fifth of those diagnosed with asthma had never received treatment for asthma in their lifetime, and smoking prevalence in those with asthma did not differ from the overall global prevalence rates for smoking.[2]

It is estimated that asthma accounts for about 1 in every 250 deaths worldwide. Many of these deaths are preventable, being attributable to suboptimal long-term medical care and delay in obtaining help during the final attack.[3] Suboptimal care for asthma can occur in highly industrialized countries, and access to care is a universal concern for asthmatics.

A systematic review of the international literature examining the prevalence of asthma has clearly shown no decline in prevalence. In addition, the prevalence of symptoms suggestive of asthma that were found in several of the studies suggests that asthma may still be increasing.[4]

ASTHMA IN THE UNITED STATES

Tracking the prevalence of asthma or the number of people at a point in time that have the disease helps in examining both the current status and asthma trends over time. The number of persons with asthma in the United States has increased by 2.9% each year from 20.3 million persons in 2001 to 25.7 million persons in 2010. Of these 25.7 million, 7.0 million were children and 18.7 million were adults. Among adults, 3.1 million people aged 65 years and older had asthma. By race, 19.1 million were white, 4.7 million were black, and 1.9 million were of other races. By ethnicity, 3.6 million were Hispanic and 22.1 million were non-Hispanic.[5]

When looking at asthma health in the United States, the measure of emergency department (ED) visits for asthma is a useful measure of poorly controlled asthma. An asthma-related ED visit is well documented in the literature as a risk factor for future asthma exacerbations. Over the period 2001 through 2009, the number of ED visits fluctuated without a clear trend. In 2009 there were 2.1 million asthma-related ED visits. ED visits provide an opportunity for providers to identify and intervene in the care of patients whose asthma is poorly controlled.

Asthma hospitalization is another useful marker in identifying high-risk patients in care. Asthma hospitalizations represent a serious adverse outcome that is considered preventable with high-quality health care, patient education, and optimal management of asthma. Hospitalization is also a marker for increased risk of future asthma exacerbations. Asthma hospitalization rates between 2001 and 2009 did not show any significant trends. In 2009 there were 479,300 hospitalizations for asthma.

The number of asthma deaths and death rates (population-based rates and risk-based rates) are compiled from the complete set of death certificates filed in the 50 states and the District of Columbia. Asthma deaths are uncommon, especially among children and young adults, but they remain a focus of preventive efforts because high-quality health care and patient education should theoretically prevent asthma-related deaths.[1] National asthma guidelines recommend early treatment and special attention to patients who are at high risk of asthma-related death.[1] Predictors of death caused by asthma include 3 or more ED visits for asthma in the past year, an asthma hospitalization or ED visit in the past month, overuse of short-acting β-agonist (short-term relief medication), a history of intubation or stay in an intensive care unit for asthma, difficulty perceiving asthma symptoms, lack of a written asthma action plan, certain patient characteristics (low socioeconomic status, female, nonwhite, current smoker, or major psychosocial problems), and the presence of other medical conditions such as cardiovascular disease.[1] The number of asthma deaths declined steadily from 2001 (4269) to 2009 (3388) at a rate of 3.3% per year.

Among patients with asthma, death rates were higher for adults (18 years and older), at a rate of 1.9 per 10,000 persons with asthma compared with 0.3 per 10,000 children with asthma.

Females (1.6 per 10,000 persons with asthma) had a greater rate than males (1.2 per 10,000 persons with asthma). The death rate for blacks (2.3 per 10,000 persons with asthma) was greater than that for whites (1.3 per 10,000 persons with asthma), and non-Hispanics (1.5 per 10,000 persons with asthma) had higher rates than Hispanics (0.9 per 10,000 persons with asthma). Although there was a decline in the death rate for all asthmatics, the disparity between races remained. The death rate per 10,000 persons with asthma for black persons was 1.6 to 2.0 times higher than the rate for white persons during each year from 2001 to 2009. The death rate for non-Hispanic persons with asthma was 1.3 to 2.0 times higher than the rate for Hispanic persons during each year.

INDOOR ENVIRONMENTAL RISK FACTORS

The role of indoor allergens and irritants is well known for its role in asthma severity as well as asthma control. The most common asthma allergens and irritants are house-dust mites, animal proteins, cockroaches, endotoxin, fungi, and smoking/environmental tobacco smoke. Improved energy efficiency of constructed and updated buildings is thought to increase exposure to allergens and respiratory irritants alongside the increase in the amount of time spent indoors in a closed space. Lifestyle and energy-efficient modifications include wall-to-wall carpeting, increased insulation, and increased indoor temperature.[6,7]

Exposure to indoor allergens is also thought to play a role in the exacerbation of asthma. Action taken to control or minimize exposure to these allergens is difficult and requires focused ongoing efforts. For example, house-dust mites are found in mattresses and bedding but also in carpets, upholstered furniture, drapes, and clothing. Dust mites absorb humidity from their surroundings, feed primarily on skin shed by humans and animals, and are commonly found in warm, humid environments.[8,9] Methods to minimize exposure to dust mites include barriers (eg, mattress and pillow covers), decreasing the humidity within rooms, and frequent vacuuming of beds, carpets, and upholstered furnishings. Dust-mite infestation is less common in high-altitude regions and arid climates, such as the mountain and Southwest regions of the United States.[10] Dust-mite fecal pellets can stimulate the immune system.[11,12] Air filtration is thought to play a limited role in controlling exposure to dust mites in undisturbed rooms. Exposure is believed to occur primarily by close proximity to sources of dust mites, such as in bed or on upholstered furniture. Exposure to dust mites was found to be an important predictor of dust-mite allergen sensitization and the development of asthma.[13]

Several investigations have suggested that exposure and sensitization to cockroach allergen may be an important factor in the development asthma in inner-city areas,[14–16] because cockroaches are ubiquitous and also highly allergenic in sensitized individuals.[17] Cockroach allergen is found in the fecal material and shed exoskeletons of cockroaches. Morbidity from asthma in inner-city children is associated with the presence of cockroach allergy and exposure to high levels of cockroach allergen found in bedroom dust.[18] Elevated levels of cockroach allergen have also been associated with urban residence, low socioeconomic status, and residence in apartment buildings in comparison with single-family homes. Exposure and sensitivity to cockroach allergen show evidence of geographic differences nationally among children who reside in the inner cities. Findings from the Inner-City Asthma Study suggest that cockroach exposure and sensitivity predominate in the humid climates of the Southern and Northeastern United States.[10]

Sensitivity and exposure to the fungus *Alternaria* is also related with asthma.[19,20] Alternata allergens are commonly found in United States households, with elevated concentrations found in the grain-growing areas of the Midwest.[21] In a representative sample of United States households, antigen levels were influenced not only by regional characteristics but also by housing and lifestyle factors. Independent predictors of *Alternaria* antigen levels were older homes, Midwest and Southern census regions, nonurban homes, low socioeconomic status, white race, mold and moisture problems, use of dehumidifier, and presence of cats and dogs. In addition, less frequent cleaning and smoking indoors increased household *Alternaria* antigen levels.[22] Using a nationally representative sample of residential homes, a large cross-sectional study found that exposure to *Alternaria* allergen in surface dust was associated with an increased risk of current asthma (physician-diagnosed asthma with asthma symptoms in the past year).[20] Damp household conditions are complex and may be confounded by other factors. In addition to mold, dampness promotes bacteria and dust-mite proliferation, and may also cause chemicals to be released from decaying furniture and building materials.[23]

Another common airway irritant, cigarette smoke, is associated with increased severity in asthma symptoms and hospitalization rates as well as a decline in lung function and an impaired response to inhaled and systemic glucocorticoids, in comparison with nonsmokers.[24–31] Smoking cessation is associated with improved lung function.[32] Smoking is an important risk factor for the development of new asthma cases and is thought to be associated with hyperresponsiveness.[33,34] Exposure to environmental smoke from tobacco exacerbates inflammatory airway responsiveness to allergens. Second-hand smoke exposure has also been associated with the development of asthma in early life,[35] with maternal smoking being the most important source of second-hand smoke exposure because of the greater exposure of children to mothers than to fathers.[36] Asthma may develop at any age, although new-onset asthma most commonly occurs in childhood.

Exposure to infectious pathogens, as well as normal gut microbiota, may influence the development of the immune system in early life. The hygiene hypothesis postulates that better hygiene, resulting in decreased microbial exposure, leads to an increase in allergic disease.[37,38]

Domesticated cats and dogs are a common source of allergens. However, an increasing number of exotic or nontraditional pets, including reptiles, birds, insects, rodents, and ferrets, have become more prevalent, and allergic responses to these animals have also been observed.[39] Cat allergen is transferred on clothing, and has been detected in schools and in houses without a cat.[17,40] Allergen concentrations detected at these sites were elevated, and in some instances this was well within concentrations of allergen found in residences with a cat or dog. Furthermore, this passively transferred allergen can become airborne and thus cause symptoms in sensitized individuals.[41,42] Exposure to cat and dog allergens during early life has been found to be both associated with and protective against the development of asthma.[35,43] Other exposures such as environmental tobacco smoke and pollution may modulate the impact of early-life exposure to animal allergen, providing a potential explanation for the variation in development of asthma.[35] Early-life exposure to farm animals was found to be negatively associated with the development of asthma and atopic sensitization.[44,45] It is not clear whether such inverse findings are due to increased exposure to allergens or increased exposure to a wide range of microbial exposures.[46]

Endotoxins are inflammatory cell-wall lipopolysaccharide molecules from gram-negative bacteria that are thought to play an important role in the development and severity of asthma,[47] although endotoxin may also be protective against atopy. Depending on the timing of exposure, household exposure to endotoxin is common.[48–50] Predictors of increased endotoxin levels, in a single study that examined collected dust samples from the living-room floor, were older buildings, lower-story residence, longer occupancy, infrequent vacuum cleaning, dog and cat ownership, and mouse infestation.[51] Other studies have negatively associated animals within the home (or joined structure) with the development of allergic disease. These animals included cats, dogs, and farm animals.[52–55] The findings would support the hygiene hypothesis proposing that exposure to microbes or germs is protective in the development of asthma, whereas clean or hygienic environments predispose one to atopy.[37,38] An association was also found between increasing endotoxin levels in bedroom and bedding dust and diagnosed asthma, asthma symptoms in the past year, current use of asthma medications, and wheezing.[47]

Epidemiologic investigations have also found associations between the development of asthma and both the use of acetaminophen and exposure to antibiotics during infancy. However, these studies have inadequately accounted for confounding bias, and warrant further investigation.[56–58]

OUTDOOR ENVIRONMENTAL RISK FACTORS

Outdoor environmental irritants, such as vehicle exhaust, can induce asthma symptoms. In addition, air pollution and desert dust can trigger symptoms in asthmatic individuals. In an investigation of reunified Germany, East Germany had consistently elevated levels of sulfur dioxide (SO_2) and other particulates, whereas West Germany had low levels of SO_2 but slightly higher levels of nitrogen dioxide (NO_2). Prevalence rates of asthma and atopic sensitization were elevated in West Germany, and bronchitis rates were elevated in East Germany. This finding is suggestive of an effect of air pollution on asthma prevalence.[59,60] Epidemiologic studies have related the exacerbation of asthma with an increase in ambient inhalable particulate matter from air pollutants, and suggest a possible role of diesel exhaust particles because inhalable particles efficiently deliver airborne allergens deep into the airways, where they can exacerbate asthma symptoms. In a prospective cohort study, onset and incidence of asthma was associated with proximity to a major roadway.[61–64] In addition, increases in ambient particulate matter, elemental carbon found in soot, NO_2, and ozone have been associated with an increase in wheezing, sales of short-acting bronchodilator medication, and increased asthma hospitalizations.[65–67] Desert dust, consisting of quartz particles also called crystalline silica, have been associated with respiratory disease in occupationally exposed individuals. Dust particles originating from desert-dust storms in one geographic location can be transported across the atmosphere to affect wide regions, and days with high concentrations of desert dust were associated with an increase in asthma hospitalizations.[68]

EMOTIONAL FACTORS

An increasing number of investigations are examining the effect on asthma of living in a violent environment. Geographic variation has been noted in asthma outcomes among large cities[69] and among neighborhoods within cities.[70–72] Exposure to community violence, explained by Wright and Steinbach[73] as proximity to violence, either through direct victimization or observing arguments, fights, or crime within neighborhoods, adds to the stressors that are likely to already burden vulnerable populations. Exposure to community violence is disproportionately experienced by low-income households, ethnic minorities, and those living within the inner city, the same groups that are also disproportionately affected by asthma.[74,75] Exposure to violence has been associated with worse control of asthma.[75] Depression, chronic stress, and stressors including exposure to community violence have been related to increased rates of asthma exacerbation in asthma patients.[73,76] Furthermore, a prospective cohort study found that caretaker depression and stress were associated with increased asthma severity in children.[77]

REFERENCES

1. National Institutes of Health National Heart Blood and Lung Institute. Guidelines for the diagnosis and management of asthma (EPR-3). Full report 2007. Bethesda (MD): National Institutes of Health National Heart Blood and Lung Institute; 2007.
2. To T, Stanojevic S, Moores G, et al. Global asthma prevalence in adults: findings from the cross-sectional world health survey. BMC Public Health 2012;12:204.
3. Masoli M, Fabian D, Holt S, et al. The global burden of asthma: executive summary of the GINA Dissemination Committee report. Allergy 2004;59:469–78.
4. Anandan C, Nurmatov U, van Schayck OC, et al. Is the prevalence of asthma declining? Systematic review of epidemiological studies. Allergy 2010;65: 152–67.
5. Akinbami LJ, Moorman JE, Bailey CM, et al. National Surveillance of Asthma: United States, 2001-2010, in National Center for Health Statistics. Vital Health Stat 3 2012;(35).
6. Platts-Mills TA. How environment affects patients with allergic disease: indoor allergens and asthma. Ann Allergy 1994;72:381–4.

7. Weiss ST, Speizer FE. Bronchial asthma mechanisms and therapeutics. In: Weiss EB, Stein M, editors. Epidemiology and natural history. Boston: Little, Brown; 1993. p. 15.
8. Spieksma FT, Dieges PH. The history of the finding of the house dust mite. J Allergy Clin Immunol 2004;113:573–6.
9. Tovey ER, Chapman MD, Wells CW, et al. The distribution of dust mite allergen in the houses of patients with asthma. Am Rev Respir Dis 1981;124:630–5.
10. Gruchalla RS, Pongracic J, Plaut M, et al. Inner city asthma study: relationships among sensitivity, allergen exposure, and asthma morbidity. J Allergy Clin Immunol 2005;115:478–85.
11. Ghaemmaghami AM, Robins A, Gough L, et al. Human T cell subset commitment determined by the intrinsic property of antigen: the proteolytic activity of the major mite allergen Der P 1 conditions T cells to produce more IL-4 and less IFN-gamma. Eur J Immunol 2001;31:1211–6.
12. Wan H, Winton HL, Soeller C, et al. Der P 1 facilitates transepithelial allergen delivery by disruption of tight junctions. J Clin Invest 1999;104:123–33.
13. Sporik R, Holgate ST, Platts-Mills TA, et al. Exposure to house-dust mite allergen (Der P I) and the development of asthma in childhood. A prospective study. N Engl J Med 1990;323:502–7.
14. Call RS, Smith TF, Morris E, et al. Risk factors for asthma in inner city children. J Pediatr 1992;121:862–6.
15. Kang B. Study on cockroach antigen as a probable causative agent in bronchial asthma. J Allergy Clin Immunol 1976;58:357–65.
16. Kang BC, Johnson J, Veres-Thorner C. Atopic profile of inner-city asthma with a comparative analysis on the cockroach-sensitive and ragweed-sensitive subgroups. J Allergy Clin Immunol 1993;92:802–11.
17. Gelber LE, Seltzer LH, Bouzoukis JK, et al. Sensitization and exposure to indoor allergens as risk factors for asthma among patients presenting to hospital. Am Rev Respir Dis 1993;147:573–8.
18. Rosenstreich DL, Eggleston P, Kattan M, et al. The role of cockroach allergy and exposure to cockroach allergen in causing morbidity among inner-city children with asthma. N Engl J Med 1997;336:1356–63.
19. Bush RK, Prochnau JJ. Alternaria-induced asthma. J Allergy Clin Immunol 2004; 113:227–34.
20. Salo PM, Arbes SJ Jr, Sever M, et al. Exposure to Alternaria alternata in US homes is associated with asthma symptoms. J Allergy Clin Immunol 2006;118:892–8.
21. O'Hollaren MT, Yunginger JW, Offord KP, et al. Exposure to an aeroallergen as a possible precipitating factor in respiratory arrest in young patients with asthma. N Engl J Med 1991;324:359–63.
22. Salo PM, Yin M, Arbes SJ Jr, et al. Dustborne Alternaria alternata antigens in US homes: results from the National survey of lead and allergens in housing. J Allergy Clin Immunol 2005;116:623–9.
23. Stokstad E. Public health. Asthma linked to indoor dampness. Science 2004;304: 1229.
24. Althuis MD, Sexton M, Prybylski D. Cigarette smoking and asthma symptom severity among adult asthmatics. J Asthma 1999;36:257–64.
25. Apostol GG, Jacobs DR Jr, Tsai AW, et al. Early life factors contribute to the decrease in lung function between ages 18 and 40: the coronary artery risk development in young adults study. Am J Respir Crit Care Med 2002;166:166–72.
26. Chalmers GW, Macleod KJ, Little SA, et al. Influence of cigarette smoking on inhaled corticosteroid treatment in mild asthma. Thorax 2002;57:226–30.

27. Chaudhuri R, Livingston E, McMahon AD, et al. Cigarette smoking impairs the therapeutic response to oral corticosteroids in chronic asthma. Am J Respir Crit Care Med 2003;168:1308–11.
28. Lange P, Parner J, Vestbo J, et al. A 15-year follow-up study of ventilatory function in adults with asthma. N Engl J Med 1998;339:1194–200.
29. Silverman RA, Boudreaux ED, Woodruff PG, et al. Cigarette smoking among asthmatic adults presenting to 64 emergency departments. Chest 2003;123: 1472–9.
30. Siroux V, Pin I, Oryszczyn MP, et al. Relationships of active smoking to asthma and asthma severity in the EGEA study. Epidemiological study on the genetics and environment of asthma. Eur Respir J 2000;15:470–7.
31. Tomlinson JE, McMahon AD, Chaudhuri R, et al. Efficacy of low and high dose inhaled corticosteroid in smokers versus non-smokers with mild asthma. Thorax 2005;60:282–7.
32. Chaudhuri R, Livingston E, McMahon AD, et al. Effects of smoking cessation on lung function and airway inflammation in smokers with asthma. Am J Respir Crit Care Med 2006;174:127–33.
33. Gilliland FD, Islam T, Berhane K, et al. Regular smoking and asthma incidence in adolescents. Am J Respir Crit Care Med 2006;174:1094–100.
34. Polosa R, Knoke JD, Russo C, et al. Cigarette smoking is associated with a greater risk of incident asthma in allergic rhinitis. J Allergy Clin Immunol 2008;121: 1428–34.
35. Carlsten C, Brauer M, Dimich-Ward H, et al. Combined exposure to dog and indoor pollution: incident asthma in a high-risk birth cohort. Eur Respir J 2011; 37:324–30.
36. Weiss KB, Gergen PJ, Wagener DK. Breathing better or wheezing worse? The changing epidemiology of asthma morbidity and mortality. Annu Rev Public Health 1993;14:491–513.
37. Fishbein AB, Fuleihan RL. The hygiene hypothesis revisited: does exposure to infectious agents protect us from allergy? Curr Opin Pediatr 2012;24:98–102.
38. Okada H, Kuhn C, Feillet H, et al. The 'hygiene hypothesis' for autoimmune and allergic diseases: an update. Clin Exp Immunol 2010;160:1–9.
39. Phillips JF, Lockey RF. Exotic pet allergy. J Allergy Clin Immunol 2009;123:513–5.
40. Custovic A, Green R, Taggart SC, et al. Domestic allergens in public places. II: dog (Can F1) and cockroach (Bla G 2) allergens in dust and mite, cat, dog and cockroach allergens in the air in public buildings. Clin Exp Allergy 1996;26: 1246–52.
41. Almqvist C, Wickman M, Perfetti L, et al. Worsening of asthma in children allergic to cats, after indirect exposure to cat at school. Am J Respir Crit Care Med 2001; 163:694–8.
42. Bollinger ME, Eggleston PA, Flanagan E, et al. Cat antigen in homes with and without cats may induce allergic symptoms. J Allergy Clin Immunol 1996;97: 907–14.
43. Kerkhof M, Wijga AH, Brunekreef B, et al. Effects of pets on asthma development up to 8 years of age: the PIAMA study. Allergy 2009;64:1202–8.
44. Braun-Fahrlander C, Riedler J, Herz U, et al, Allergy, and Team Endotoxin Study. Environmental exposure to endotoxin and its relation to asthma in school-age children. N Engl J Med 2002;347:869–77.
45. Illi S, Depner M, Genuneit J, et al, Gabriela Study Group. Protection from childhood asthma and allergy in alpine farm environments—the Gabriel advanced studies. J Allergy Clin Immunol 2012;129:1470–1477.e6.

46. Ege MJ, Mayer M, Normand AC, et al, Gabriela Transregio 22 Study Group. Exposure to environmental microorganisms and childhood asthma. N Engl J Med 2011;364:701–9.
47. Thorne PS, Kulhankova K, Yin M, et al. Endotoxin exposure is a risk factor for asthma: the national survey of endotoxin in United States housing. Am J Respir Crit Care Med 2005;172:1371–7.
48. Michel O, Kips J, Duchateau J, et al. Severity of asthma is related to endotoxin in house dust. Am J Respir Crit Care Med 1996;154:1641–6.
49. Modig L, Toren K, Janson C, et al. Vehicle exhaust outside the home and onset of asthma among adults. Eur Respir J 2009;33:1261–7.
50. Park JH, Spiegelman DL, Burge HA, et al. Longitudinal study of dust and airborne endotoxin in the home. Environ Health Perspect 2000;108:1023–8.
51. Bischof W, Koch A, Gehring U, et al, Exposure Indoor, and Group Genetics in Asthma Study. Predictors of high endotoxin concentrations in the settled dust of German homes. Indoor Air 2002;12:2–9.
52. Hesselmar B, Aberg N, Aberg B, et al. Does early exposure to cat or dog protect against later allergy development? Clin Exp Allergy 1999;29:611–7.
53. Ownby DR, Johnson CC, Peterson EL. Exposure to dogs and cats in the first year of life and risk of allergic sensitization at 6 to 7 years of age. JAMA 2002;288:963–72.
54. Platts-Mills TA, Perzanowski M, Woodfolk JA, et al. Relevance of early or current pet ownership to the prevalence of allergic disease. Clin Exp Allergy 2002;32:335–8.
55. Platts-Mills T, Vaughan J, Squillace S, et al. Sensitisation, asthma, and a modified Th2 response in children exposed to cat allergen: a population-based cross-sectional study. Lancet 2001;357:752–6.
56. Beasley R, Clayton T, Crane J, et al, ISAAC Phase Three Study Group. Association between paracetamol use in infancy and childhood, and risk of asthma, rhinoconjunctivitis, and eczema in children aged 6-7 years: analysis from Phase Three of the ISAAC programme. Lancet 2008;372(9643):1039.
57. McKeever TM, Lewis SA, Smit HA, et al. The association of acetaminophen, aspirin, and ibuprofen with respiratory disease and lung function. Am J Respir Crit Care Med 2005;171(9):966.
58. Marra F, Lynd L, Coombes M, et al. Does antibiotic exposure during infancy lead to development of asthma?: a systematic review and metaanalysis. Chest 2006;129(3):610.
59. Magnussen H, Jorres R, Nowak D. Effect of air pollution on the prevalence of asthma and allergy: lessons from the German reunification. Thorax 1993;48:879–81.
60. von Mutius E, Martinez FD, Fritzsch C, et al. Prevalence of asthma and atopy in two areas of West and East Germany. Am J Respir Crit Care Med 1994;149:358–64.
61. Bleck B, Tse DB, Jaspers I, et al. Diesel exhaust particle-exposed human bronchial epithelial cells induce dendritic cell maturation. J Immunol 2006;176:7431–7.
62. Boland S, Baeza-Squiban A, Fournier T, et al. Diesel exhaust particles are taken up by human airway epithelial cells in vitro and alter cytokine production. Am J Physiol 1999;276:L604–13.
63. Jin C, Shelburne CP, Li G, et al. Particulate allergens potentiate allergic asthma in mice through sustained IgE-mediated mast cell activation. J Clin Invest 2011;121:941–55.

64. Ohtoshi T, Takizawa H, Okazaki H, et al. Diesel exhaust particles stimulate human airway epithelial cells to produce cytokines relevant to airway inflammation in vitro. J Allergy Clin Immunol 1998;101:778–85.
65. Kanatani KT, Ito I, Al-Delaimy WK, et al, Dust Toyama Asian Desert, and Team Asthma Study. Desert dust exposure is associated with increased risk of asthma hospitalization in children. Am J Respir Crit Care Med 2010;182:1475–81.
66. Roy A, Sheffield P, Wong K, et al. The effects of outdoor air pollutants on the costs of pediatric asthma hospitalizations in the United States, 1999 to 2007. Med Care 2011;49:810–7.
67. Spira-Cohen A, Chen LC, Kendall M, et al. Personal exposures to traffic-related air pollution and acute respiratory health among Bronx schoolchildren with asthma. Environ Health Perspect 2011;119:559–65.
68. Laurent O, Pedrono G, Filleul L, et al. Influence of socioeconomic deprivation on the relation between air pollution and beta-agonist sales for asthma. Chest 2009; 135:717–23.
69. Perrin JM, Homer CJ, Berwick DM, et al. Variations in rates of hospitalization of children in three urban communities. N Engl J Med 1989;320:1183–7.
70. Carr W, Zeitel L, Weiss K. Variations in asthma hospitalizations and deaths in New York city. Am J Public Health 1992;82:59–65.
71. Lang DM, Polansky M. Patterns of asthma mortality in Philadelphia from 1969 to 1991. N Engl J Med 1994;331:1542–6.
72. Marder D, Targonski P, Orris P, et al. Effect of racial and socioeconomic factors on asthma mortality in Chicago. Chest 1992;101:426S–9S.
73. Wright RJ, Steinbach SF. Violence: an unrecognized environmental exposure that may contribute to greater asthma morbidity in high risk inner-city populations. Environ Health Perspect 2001;109:1085–9.
74. Clark C, Ryan L, Kawachi I, et al. Witnessing community violence in residential neighborhoods: a mental health hazard for urban women. J Urban Health 2008; 85:22–38.
75. Wright RJ, Mitchell H, Visness CM, et al. Community violence and asthma morbidity: the inner-city asthma study. Am J Public Health 2004;94:625–32.
76. Apter AJ, Garcia LA, Boyd RC, et al. Exposure to community violence is associated with asthma hospitalizations and emergency department visits. J Allergy Clin Immunol 2010;126:552–7.
77. Wright RJ, Cohen S, Carey V, et al. Parental stress as a predictor of wheezing in infancy: a prospective birth-cohort study. Am J Respir Crit Care Med 2002;165: 358–65.

Pathophysiology, Diagnosis, and Clinical Assessment of Asthma in the Adult

Kathryn Killeen, MSN, APN, ACNP-BC, CCNS[a],*,
Elizabeth Skora, MSN, APN, ANP-BC[b]

KEYWORDS

• Adult • Asthma • Pathophysiology • Diagnosis • Assessment • Treatment

KEY POINTS

- A thorough review of medical history coupled with confirmatory diagnostic testing is essential to the diagnosis of asthma.
- Spirometry continues to be the first-line testing as recommended by the Global Initiative for Asthma and The Expert Panel Report 3.
- Bronchial challenge testing, by either methacholine or mannitol, can be useful in assessing airway hyperresponsiveness in the setting of normal spirometry.
- When added with other clinical data, the evaluation of fractional exhaled nitric oxide may be helpful in the diagnosis of asthma; but further research is needed to evaluate its utility in the management of asthma.
- All efforts should be made to bolster early diagnosis and evaluation of asthma in an effort to achieve optimal control of asthma symptoms and to minimize airway inflammation, hyperresponsiveness, and remodeling.

Asthma is a chronic inflammatory disorder that is characterized by 3 distinct responses: pulmonary inflammation, airway hyperresponsiveness, and airway remodeling in response to a host of triggers that affect only those who are predisposed to the disease. These responses can vary widely not only among individuals but also over time. The key factors that determine the presence and extent of disease severity include the time of disease presentation and/or diagnosis as well as the persistence of illness.[1] Clinical diagnosis of asthma is often based on the presence of symptoms,

Funding sources: None.
Conflict of interest: None.
[a] The Division of Pulmonary and Critical Care Medicine, Department of Adult Critical Care Nursing, Rush University Medical Center, 1725 West Harrison, Suite 054, Chicago, IL 60612, USA; [b] Department of Adult and Gerontological Nursing, Rush University College of Nursing, 600 South Paulina Street, Suite 1053, Chicago, IL 60612, USA
* Corresponding author.
E-mail address: Kathryn_M_Killeen@rush.edu

such as cough, wheeze, breathlessness, and chest tightness; but the presence of these symptoms is not exclusive to asthma, and clinical correlation with spirometry and other diagnostic testing is essential. This article presents a review of current literature and discusses the pathophysiology, diagnosis, and clinical assessment of asthma in the adult patient population. The authors discuss current standards for the assessment and diagnosis.

EPIDEMIOLOGY AND RISK FACTORS

From 2001 to 2009, the number of people diagnosed with asthma grew by 4.3 million. Asthma costs in the United States grew from approximately 6% from 2002 to 2007, approximately $53 billion and $56 billion, respectively.[2] Based on a recent National Center for Health Statistics data brief in 2012, asthma prevalence increased from 7.3% in 2001 to 8.4% in 2010. In 2010, it has been estimated that 25.7 million persons had asthma: 18.7 million adults (aged $\geq$18 years) and 17.0 million children (aged 0–17 years). Furthermore, asthma mortality seems to be higher for females, black individuals, and adults. From 2007 to 2009, the asthma death rate per 1000 persons with asthma was 0.15. Asthma death rates per 1000 persons with asthma were more than 30% higher for females than males, 75% higher for the black population than the white population, and almost 7 times higher for adults than children.[3]

Factors that influence the risk of asthma can be differentiated into 2 separate categories: host factors that cause the development of asthma and environmental factors that trigger asthma symptoms. In some cases, a factor can do both.[4] A summary of the factors that influence the development and expression of asthma can be found in **Box 1**. Obesity (body mass index >30 kg/m^2) is not only strongly linked to an increased

---

Box 1
Factors influencing the development and expression of asthma GINA

Host factors

  Genetic

    Genes predisposing to atopy

    Genes predisposing to airway hyperresponsiveness

  Obesity

  Sex

Environmental factors

  Allergens

    Indoor: domestic mites, furred animals (dogs, cats, mice), cockroach allergen, fungi, molds, yeasts

    Outdoor: pollens, fungi, molds, yeasts

  Infections (predominantly viral)

  Occupational sensitizers

  Tobacco smoke

  Outdoor/indoor air pollution

  Diet

From the Global Strategy for Asthma Management and Prevention, 2012 used with permission from the Global Initiative for Asthma (GINA), www.ginasthma.org.

risk of asthma but also poor control. Obese individuals have poorer lung function and more comorbidities as compared with normal-weight people with asthma. How obesity promotes asthma development is still uncertain; but there are many hypotheses, including the effect on the mechanics of lung function, the development of a proinflammatory state, and other hormonal influences.[4,5] In addition, age seems to be a critical factor. Males have an increased prevalence of asthma before the age of 14 years; but at puberty, the prevalence of asthma is greater in females.[4,6] Diet has also been identified as a factor. Breastfeeding in particular has been an area of study whereby it was proved that infants who were fed formula rather than breast milk have a higher incidence of wheezing illnesses. In addition, some characteristics of Western diets, including an increase in processed foods and a decrease in antioxidant-rich foods (ie, fruits and vegetables), also have contributed to asthma and other atopic disease.[4] Lastly, although there is information linking several respiratory viruses during infancy with an associated increased risk of asthma, there are also those individuals who think that the exposure to certain infections early in life may protect against asthma development; this is referred to as the *hygiene hypothesis* of asthma. This hypothesis suggests that exposure to infections early in life influences the development of a child's immune system along a nonallergic pathway, therefore, leading to a reduced risk of asthma and other allergic diseases.[4–6]

DEFINITION AND PATHOPHYSIOLOGY

National and international guidelines aimed to strategize efforts for the management and prevention of asthma have been published. The Expert Panel Report 3 (EPR 3) published in 2007 from the National Heart, Lung, and Blood Institute has been considered to be one of the leading references on the topic of the diagnosis and treatment of asthma. Another such initiative is the Global Initiative for Asthma (GINA) revised in 2011.[4] GINA describes asthma as a disorder that is characterized by its clinical, physiologic, and pathologic characteristics. The 2011 GINA guidelines define asthma as follows:

> *Asthma is a chronic inflammatory disorder of the airways in which many cells and cellular elements play a role. The chronic inflammation is associated with airway hyperresponsiveness that leads to recurrent episodes of wheezing, breathlessness, chest tightness, and coughing, particularly at night or in the early morning. These episodes are usually associated with widespread, but variable airflow obstruction within the lung that is often reversible either spontaneously or with treatment.[4(p16)]*

The pathogenesis of asthma is not yet clearly understood; as a result, much of the definition of asthma is descriptive. As further research develops, we continue to learn more about the inflammatory cells and mediators that may be the key to minimizing the frequency and severity of asthma exacerbations.

AIRWAY INFLAMMATION AND AIRWAY HYPERRESPONSIVENESS

Airway inflammation is the hallmark of the development of asthma and the pathophysiology of the disease. Inflammation occurs as a result of infiltration of numerous inflammatory mediators to the area. The level of inflammation determines the severity, frequency, and extent of illness in patients with asthma.[6] Exposure to causative agents triggers an immune-mediated response in susceptible individuals, setting off an inflammatory cascade with a variable degree of airway obstruction. This reaction is a multifactorial process, which involves the participation of various cell types in the tissues of the respiratory tract as well as other organ systems, including the bone marrow and lymphoid, vascular, and nervous systems.[1] Airway inflammation is persistent in the disease, although symptoms may be episodic.[4] There are numerous inflammatory cells found in asthmatic airways, the majority in increased quantity. Some of these include lymphocytes, mast cells, eosinophils, neutrophils, dendritic cells, and macrophages. All of these release mediators that contribute to the inflammation, which is the cornerstone of disease expression.[4]

Airway hyperresponsiveness (AHR) occurs directly in conjunction with airway inflammation and is also characteristic of asthma. AHR is the contraction of small muscles surrounding the airways, which limits a person's ability to more freely move air throughout the lungs. Exposure to causative agents (ie, triggers), including exercise, infection (viral), environmental allergens (house dust mites, pollen, cat dander), occupational exposures (chemicals), airborne irritants (tobacco smoke), strong odors, cold air, and other inhaled irritants,[1,3,4,7] activates an immune-mediated response, which is further discussed later and is illustrated in **Fig. 1**. Exposure can lead to recurrent episodes of wheezing, breathlessness, chest tightness, and coughing, particularly at night or in the early morning.[7]

INFLAMMATORY CELLS
Lymphocytes

Lymphocytes have 2 subpopulations: T helper 1 (Th1) cells and T helper 2 (Th2) cells, which have distinct inflammatory mediator profiles and effects on airway function.[6] T lymphocytes aggregate in asthmatic airways and release inflammatory mediators, cytokines (interleukin [IL]-4, IL-5, IL-9, and IL-13) that stimulate eosinophilic inflammation and B lymphocytic production of immunoglobulin E (IgE). Elevated levels of IgE, also known as atopy, are associated with a Th2 lymphocyte-driven immune response.[1,4] It is thought that the increased activity of Th2 lymphocytes is partly caused by a reduction of regulatory T cells that normally inhibit these cells.[4]

Mast Cells

Mast cells release bronchoconstrictor mediators, such as histamine, cysteinyl leukotrienes, and prostaglandin D_2, which lead to AHR.[4,6] These cells are activated by 2 main mechanisms: first, activation through high-affinity IgE receptors and second, osmotic stimuli (ie, exercise-induced bronchoconstriction).[4] The mast cell has large numbers of IgE receptors. When activated by the interaction with an antigen, these release a wide variety of mediators that initiate bronchospasm and also release proinflammatory cytokines to bring about airway inflammation. IgE is the antibody largely responsible for the activation of allergic reactions and is key to the pathogenesis of allergic diseases and the development and persistence of inflammation.[1,6]

Eosinophils

Eosinophils are the prominent cells in the airways of most, but not all, patients with asthma.[5,6] An increase in numbers often correlates with increased asthma severity. The aggregation of these cells is common in the blood, bone marrow, and lung, which has lead to the belief that the eosinophil is the central effector cell in asthma that contributes to ongoing inflammation.[5] In addition, eosinophils are thought to release basic proteins that may damage airway epithelial cells and may also have a role in the release of growth factors and airway remodeling.[4]

Neutrophils

Neutrophils are increased in the airways and sputum of patients with severe asthma, during acute exacerbations, and in smokers. The pathophysiologic role of these cells

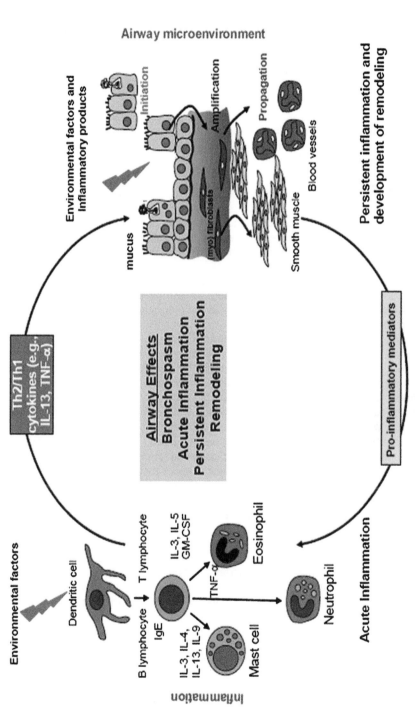

Fig. 1. Factors limiting airflow in acute and persistent asthma. GM-CSF, granulocyte-macrophage colony-stimulating factor; IgE, immunoglobulin E; IL-3, interleukin 3 (and similar); Th, T helper; TNF-α, tumor necrosis factor-alpha. (*From* Holgate ST, Polosa R. The mechanisms, diagnosis, and management of severe asthma in adults. Lancet 2006;368(9537):780–93.)

is not well understood. Some think that their increase in number may be caused by glucosteroid use.[4,6]

Dendritic Cells

Dendritic cells interact with allergens from the airway surface and then migrate to regional lymph nodes to interact with regulatory cells that ultimately stimulate Th2 cell production.[6]

Macrophages

Macrophages are abundant in airways and are thought to be activated by allergens through IgE receptors to release inflammatory mediators and cytokines, which amplify the inflammatory response.[4,6]

INFLAMMATORY MEDIATORS
Chemokines

Chemokines recruit inflammatory cells into the airways and are mainly expressed in the airway epithelial cells.[4,6] There is increasing data linking the role of chemokines in the activation of injury, as it relates to the pathophysiology of asthma.[6]

Cytokines

Cytokines orchestrate the inflammatory response in asthma and determine its severity. Th2 cytokines regulate allergic inflammation via the production of IL-3, IL-4, IL-5, IL-9, IL-10, and IL-13.[1,4,5]

IL-4 is critical for the synthesis of IgE and is involved in eosinophil recruitment to the airways. It is also crucial in Th2 cell differentiation and, therefore, is currently being investigated as a potential site for inhibition in the treatment of asthma. Similarly, IL-13 is also needed for IgE formation in fact, it has been suggested that there must be sufficient IL-13 levels in order to induce allergic asthma. When present in increased amounts, typical asthma characteristics become more apparent, including AHR, eosinophilia, mucus hypersecretion, and subepithelial fibrosis.[5] Both IL-4 and IL-13 can influence some structure remodeling changes seen in chronic asthma. These changes include mucus hypersecretion and goblet cell metaphase.[1]

IL-5 is required for eosinophilic differentiation and survival. As a result, it has an essential role regulating eosinophilic inflammation in asthma and subsequent AHR. IL-9 is a mediator for Th2 leukocyte-driven inflammation, mast cell release, IgE production, and mucus hypersecretion. IL-10 is an antiinflammatory cytokine and acts to inhibit inflammatory cytokine expression.[1,4,5]

Cysteinyl Leukotrienes

Cysteinyl leukotrienes are mainly derived from mast cells and eosinophils. These cells are potent bronchoconstrictors and proinflammatory mediators. To date, these are the only mediators in which their inhibition has been associated with an improvement in lung function and asthma symptoms.[4,6]

Histamine

Histamine is released from mast cells and contributes to the inflammatory response, in addition to bronchoconstriction.[4]

Nitric Oxide

Nitric oxide (NO), a potent vasodilator, is produced largely by the action of inducible NO synthase in the airway epithelial cells; its presence in the airways is associated with the presence of inflammation in asthma. NO may contribute to airway narrowing by promoting vasodilatation, increased blood flow, and airway edema. Therefore, concentrations of NO found in the expired air of patients with asthma may be the result of inflammation rather than the cause.[1] Investigations are ongoing in the use of measurements of fractional exhaled NO (FeNO) in the management and diagnosis of asthma.[4–6]

Prostaglandin D₂

Prostaglandin D_2 is a bronchoconstrictor originating primarily from mast cells and is involved in Th2 cell recruitment to the airways.[4]

AIRWAY REMODELING

Airway remodeling is one of the chief pathologic features of chronic asthma[5] and is simply defined as a structural change in the bronchial tissues.[1] Recent evidence shows that remodeling may not be entirely caused by inflammation; despite the use of antiinflammatory treatments, there has been limited efficacy in the reduction of remodeling.[5]

Typical characteristics of airway remodeling found in patients with chronic, poorly controlled asthma include hyperinflation of the lungs, smooth muscle hyperplasia, basement membrane thickening, mucous gland hyperplasia, mucosal epithelial sloughing, and tissue edema.[1] Airway smooth muscle mass is increased in individuals with asthma, which contributes to a narrowing of the airway lumen. In addition, a characteristic feature of asthma is the thickening of the basal lamina beneath a normal-appearing epithelial basement membrane. The mechanisms for basement membrane thickening are, at this time, unknown and further analysis is needed. Better understood is goblet cell hyperplasia, which is a hallmark of pathologic conditions in all levels of severity of asthma, including mild, moderate, and severe disease. Under normal circumstances, mucin is secreted by goblet cells in the airway epithelium. This mucus forms a thin lining and functions in protecting the lung tissue by trapping foreign debris, bacteria, and viruses and then working with the cilia to clear captured material. In asthma, there is an excessive production of mucus, which contributes to airway obstruction. In addition, patients with asthma have a significant increase in the number of mucus-secreting goblet cells as compared with normal individuals.[5]

DIAGNOSIS

Recommendations from the EPR 3 guideline for the components necessary to the diagnosis of asthma are summarized in **Box 2**.

MEDICAL HISTORY

A thorough medical history is an essential component because the initial diagnosis of asthma is often based on the symptoms and response to prescribed therapy (eg, bronchodilators and/or inhaled glucocorticoids steroids).[6] Patients present most commonly with symptoms of cough, shortness of breath, wheezing, and chest tightness. Efforts should be made to identify precipitating or aggravating factors that might lead to symptoms. Examples of these include factors but are not limited to recent viral illness, exposure to cigarette smoke, strong scents, and hot or cold air. It is important to establish patterns of when symptoms occur because this will also provide useful data. Nighttime awakenings caused by symptoms are suggestive of asthma because of the diurnal variation of the disease. Symptoms of asthma are usually variable as opposed to

---

Box 2
Key points: diagnosis of asthma EPR 3 report (2007)

- To establish a diagnosis of asthma, the clinician should determine that (EPR 2, 1997)
  - Episodic symptoms of airflow obstruction or AHR are present
  - Airflow obstruction is at least partially reversible
  - Alternative diagnoses are excluded
- Recommended methods to establish the diagnosis are (EPR 2, 1997)
  - Detailed medical history
  - Physical examination focusing on the upper reparatory tract, chest, and skin
  - Spirometry to demonstrate obstruction and assess reversibility, including in children 5 years of age or older; reversibility determined either by an increased in forced expiratory volume in the first second of expiration (FEV_1) of 12% or more from baseline or by an increase of 10% or more of predicated FEV_1 after inhalation of a short-acting bronchodilator
  - Additional studies as necessary to exclude alternate diagnoses

From National Asthma Education and Prevention Program. Expert panel report 3 (ERP-3): Guidelines for the diagnosis and management of asthma - Full report 2007, NIH Publication Number 08-5846. 2007. p. 1–74. Available at: http://www.nhlbi.nih.gov/guidelines/asthma/asthsumm.pdf. Accessed August 9, 2012.

---

constant, which may suggest a different diagnosis (ie, chronic obstructive pulmonary disease [COPD]). However, patients in the midst of an exacerbation and/or poorly controlled asthma may also present in this manner. A review of any known allergies (ie, environmental, foods) should be completed due to the strong association of these factors with asthma. Seasonal variation in signs and symptoms, suggestive of allergies, is also important to note and will be useful in the future management of the disease. A review of patients' current medication can also provide useful data because some medications are known to cause cough (eg, angiotensin-converting enzyme [ACE] inhibitors). In patients presenting with symptoms who also have a history of nasal polyps in conjunction with aspirin sensitivity, a diagnosis of asthma should be strongly considered. This is also known as Sampter's triad. Employment history should be reviewed because it is reported that 1 out of 10 cases of asthma in working-age adults can be associated with occupational exposures.[4] Common occupations with known exposures include bakers (flour), painters (isocyanates, aldehyde), farming, plastic manufacturing, and housekeeping.[4] A review of social history should include smoking history. Although smoking is usually associated with COPD, individuals with asthma may experience deleterious effects on lung function. Some of these effects include a decline in lung function, increase in severity, decrease in effectiveness of medications, and reduction in control.[4]

Cough variant asthma should be considered when patients present with an isolated complaint of cough without other signs or suggestive triggers.[6,8] However, in individuals with an isolated cough, the possibility of gastroesophageal reflux disease (GERD) and/or upper airway cough syndromes (UAC) (previously known as postnasal drip syndrome) must also be considered.[8] Patients complaining of shortness of breath and/or wheezing only when active should be evaluated for exercise-induced asthma (EIA) using appropriate testing.[4]

Despite having a history that is suggestive of asthma, it is important to consider other potential diagnoses that have similar symptoms and presentation. Conditions with symptoms that might be similar are listed in **Box 3**. COPD is usually associated with older patients, with a history of tobacco use or exposure. Complaints of dyspnea and/or wheezing can be found in heart failure.

PHYSICAL EXAMINATION

A focused physical examination in the evaluation of asthma should include the upper respiratory tract, chest, and skin.[4,6] Pale, swollen nasal mucosa may suggest allergic rhinitis, which has an association with asthma. The observance of nasal polyps (gray, mucoid masses) may be noted (component of Sampter's triad). Cobblestoning in the posterior pharynx is consistent with postnasal drainage and known to cause asthma symptoms (ie, cough).[8] Auscultatory lung examination might be completely normal. Wheezing, usually expiratory, can be noted in any of the lung fields but cannot be used as a reliable indicator of limitation in airflow.[6] In some patients, wheezing might only be noted during forced exhalation.[6] Prolonged inspiratory to expiratory ratio and/or use of accessory muscles are usually found in patients who are experiencing moderate-severe respiratory distress caused by the disease.[9] Findings of upper airway sounds (ie, throat) are not consistent with asthma and suggest alternative diagnosis (ie, vocal cord dysfunction [VCD]). Visual inspection of the skin is valuable to assess for atopic dermatitis or eczema, both having an association with asthma.[7]

SPIROMETRY

Spirometry testing provides the ability to obtain objective measurements of lung function demonstrating the presence of airway obstruction with reversibility.[4] The EPR 3 guideline states, "Spirometry is an essential objective measure to establish the diagnosis of asthma, because the medical history and physical examination are not reliable

---

Box 3
Differential diagnosis of asthma

COPD

Congestive heart failure

Pulmonary embolism

UAC

GERD

Vocal cord dysfunction

Cystic fibrosis

Malignancy obstruction of the airways

Pulmonary infiltration with eosinophilia

Cough secondary to drugs (ie, ACE)

Allergic bronchopulmonary aspergillosis

Churg-Strauss syndrome

Data from National Asthma Education and Prevention Program. Expert panel report 3 (ERP-3): Guidelines for the diagnosis and management of asthma - Full report 2007, NIH Publication Number 08-5846. 2007. p. 1–74. Available at: http://www.nhlbi.nih.gov/guidelines/asthma/asthsumm.pdf. Accessed August 9, 2012; and McCormack M, Enright PL. Making the diagnosis of asthma. Respir Care 2008;53(5):583–92.

means of excluding other diagnosis or of assessing lung states".[6] Spirometry should be performed by trained individuals in a laboratory that that is adherent to quality-control measures, such as calibration and maintenance of testing equipment, to ensure the accuracy of the data collected.[10] In this test, patients are instructed to perform a forced exhalation maneuver, allowing for measurement of forced vital capacity (FVC) and forced expiratory volume in the first second (FEV_1) values by which a FEV_1/FVC ratio is calculated. Obstruction is identified if this ratio is less than normal (less than 75% in adults).[4] Results are compared with reference of established normal values, which are based on age, sex, height, and ethnicity (ie, National Health and Nutrition Examination Study). After the administration of a short-acting bronchodilator via a multi-dose inhaler, testing is repeated to evaluate for reversibility. An increase of 200 mL from the baseline value AND 12% indicates reversibility. These results, when combined with symptoms and history, confirm a diagnosis of asthma.

ASSESSMENT OF AHR

In patients with normal spirometry and a strong clinical suspicion, evaluation of AHR should be performed by way of bronchial challenge testing. This testing can be achieved by exposing the airways to a stimulant (ie, direct, indirect, or via exercise), causing airways to react, resulting in decreased flow in the airways. Direct stimuli, such as methacholine, work directly on the smooth muscle in the airways, causing constriction. Indirect methods expose the airways to an irritant, causing the release of endogenous mediators (ie, prostaglandins, histamine), leading to smooth muscle contraction.[11] Thresholds for maximum exposure dose to induce reaction in the airways are established. Spirometry is performed before exposure and following each exposure. A reduction in the FEV_1 (>20% for methacholine, >15% mannitol) is significant for AHR.[9,12] Testing is sensitive for asthma but not specific to the disease because hyperresponsiveness can be seen in other diseases (eg, cystic fibrosis, bronchiectasis).[4,11] Conversely, if no significant change is noted (ie, negative test), then results can be useful in excluding asthma as a diagnosis because there is no objective evidence of AHR. The option for stimulants was relatively limited to methacholine until recently when mannitol was approved by the Food and Drug Administration. Although each form of testing has its advantages and disadvantages, there are no data to support one being superior over the other in provoking a response.[12] Exercise challenge testing should be performed in individuals who experience symptoms with activity. Using a treadmill or stationary bike for up to 30 minutes, the patients' FEV_1 is evaluated at a regular interval for change at regular intervals as the grade or resistance are increased. A 10% decrease in the FEV_1 is considered diagnostic of EIA.[9]

PEAK EXPIRATORY FLOW MONITORING

Using peak expiratory flow (PEF) measurements can be helpful in the management of the disease but are not generally recommended over spirometry for use in the diagnosis of asthma because of the wide variability in peak flow meter and reference values.[6,13] Using a handheld device (ie, PEF meter), patients forcefully exhale the volume of air in their lungs, after which a measurement is obtained. PEF meters are inexpensive and provide the option of assessing lung function objectively.[4] Effective patient education is vital to proper use of PEF meters because the accuracy of the data obtained depends on the patients' effort and technique. The use of the PEF meters can be helpful in assessing patients' daily variability and improve control, particularly in patients who might under recognize asthma symptoms and severity.[4]

FURTHER TESTING
Additional Pulmonary Function Testing

Flow volume loops, obtained during spirometry graphically depict the rate of inspiratory and expiratory airflow. These loops can provide information with differentiating between asthma (scooped out appearance in expiratory limb) as opposed to findings consistent with VCD, when the defect is noted in the inspiratory portion of the curve.[13] Diffusion capacity can assist in differentiating between asthma (normal) and COPD (reduced).[13]

Chest Radiography/Chest Tomography

Chest radiography or chest tomography may be done during the workup for asthma but usually to rule out other disorders (ie, masses, parenchymal changes, cystic fibrosis).[9] In patients with asthma, chest radiography often will be normal but might reveal hyperinflation in poorly controlled asthma or during an exacerbation.

Biomarkers: Sputum Eosinophils, Fractional Exhaled Nitric Oxide Measurement

Evaluating sputum for eosinophils, markers of allergic inflammation, can be done as part of the diagnosis and assessment of asthma. Limitations of this testing include challenges in sputum collection (if induction is needed) and inconsistencies with sample analysis,[6,13] suggesting the most appropriate use of this test is in the clinical research setting.[13] Fractional exhaled nitric oxide (FeNO) is another biomarker that can also be used to assess eosinophilic airway inflammation. Advantages to FeNO testing are that it is noninvasive, delivers quantifiable results, and it is easy to use in patients with severe airway obstruction.[14] However, current testing modalities are expensive, with limited availability; the use of the data collected currently is recommended only in specific instances.[14] The use of glucocorticoids can affect levels of FeNO, leaving the full use of the testing in question because these medications are the cornerstone treatment of this disease.[4] Elevated FeNO levels are not exclusive to asthma because similar results have been found in eczema, allergic rhinitis and atopy.[15] The tests utility has proven most valuable when used to compliment other data in the diagnosis for asthma and the likelihood of untreated (ie, steroid naive) patients' response to steroids.[14] Further research is needed to ascertain how results of testing can be fully used in the management of this disease.

Allergy Testing

Given the strong association between asthma and allergic rhinitis, the presence of other allergic manifestations (atopy, elevated IgE, positive skin test) increase the likelihood of asthma in symptomatic patients.[4,13] Skin prick testing can be performed observing for skin changes (wheal and flare) after common known allergens are inserted into the skin.[13] Advantages to this testing are that it is relatively inexpensive and can be done in the office of a trained health care provider, with immediate results with high sensitivity.[4] However, improper technique can lead to inaccurate results.[4] Evaluating patients' serum IgE is another testing option. The results may reveal elevated levels that can be seen in patients who are atopic. These results must be associated with a known exposure because some patients may have an elevated IgE without symptoms.[4] Serum IgE testing is expensive and does not provide any superiority in sensitivity when compared with skin prick testing when determining allergic status.[4]

THE NEXT STEP: ASTHMA CONTROL

Once a diagnosis of asthma is established, the goal of treatment should be to achieve and maintain control of symptoms, maintain awareness of the safety and potential

Table 1
Assessment of asthma control

Characteristic	Controlled (All of the Following)	Partly Controlled (Any Measure Present in Any Week)	Uncontrolled
1. Assessment of current clinical control (over the past 4 wk)			
Daytime symptoms	None (twice or less per wk)	More than twice per wk	3 or more features of partly controlled asthma present in any wk[a,b]
Limitation of activities	None	Any	
Nocturnal symptoms/ awakening	None	Any	
Need for reliever/ rescue treatment	None (twice or less per wk)	More than twice per wk	
Lung function (PEF or FEV_1)[c]	Normal	<80% predicted or personal best (if known)	
2. Assessment of future risk (risk of exacerbations[a], instability, rapid decline in lung function, side effects)			
Patients with any of the following features are at increased risk of adverse events in the future: poor clinical control, frequent exacerbations in past year, ever admitted to critical care for asthma, low FEV_1, exposure to cigarette smoke, high-dose medication requirement			

[a] Any exacerbation should prompt review of maintenance treatment to ensure that it is adequate.
[b] By definition, an exacerbation in any week makes that an uncontrolled week.
[c] Lung function is not a reliable test for children 5 years of age and younger.
From Global Strategy for Asthma Management and Prevention, Global Initiative for Asthma (GINA) 2011. Available at: http://www.ginasthma.org/; with permission.

side effects of medication, coupled with thoughtful consideration of the costs associated with care.[4] The evaluation of control includes the assessment of patients' clinical symptoms along with the evaluation for future risk, including exacerbations, instability, side effect of medication, and decline in lung function.[4] **Table 1** represents a tool that can be used in the assessment of control as recommended by GINA. The assessment of control is imperative to effectively treat this disease with medications, whether escalating or de-escalating therapy. Good control has been shown overall to reduce the risk of exacerbations.[4]

SUMMARY

A thorough review of medical history coupled with confirmatory diagnostic testing is essential to the diagnosis of asthma. Spirometry continues to be the first-line testing as recommended by GINA and EPR 3.[4,6] Bronchial challenge testing, by either methacholine or mannitol, can be useful in assessing AHR in the setting of normal spirometry. When added with other clinical data, the evaluation of FeNO may be helpful in the diagnosis of asthma; but further research is needed to evaluate its utility in the management of asthma. All efforts should be made to bolster the early diagnosis and evaluation of asthma in an effort to achieve optimal control of asthma symptoms and to minimize airway inflammation, hyperresponsiveness, and remodeling.

REFERENCES

1. Fireman P. Understanding asthma pathophysiology. Allergy Asthma Proc 2003; 24(2):79–83.
2. CDC vital signs. Asthma in the US growing every year. 2012. Available at: http://www.cdc.gov/vitalsigns/Asthma/. Accessed August 9, 2012.
3. Akinbami LJ, Moorman JE, Bailey C, et al. Trends in asthma prevalence, health care use, and mortality in the United States, 2001-2010. NCHS data brief, no 94. Hyattsville (MD): National Center for Health Statistics; 2012.
4. Global strategy for asthma management and prevention, global initiative for asthma (GINA) 2011. Available at: http://www.ginasthma.org/.
5. Lugogo N, Loretta G, Fertel D, et al. Murray & Nadel's textbook of respiratory medicine. 5th edition. Philadelphia: Saunders; 2010. p. 883–918.
6. Summary report 2007. National asthma education and prevention program expert panel report 3: guidelines for the diagnosis and management of asthma. Available at: http://www.nhlbi.nih.gov/guidelines/asthma/asthsumm.pdf. Accessed August 9, 2012.
7. Kaufman G. Asthma: pathophysiology, diagnosis and management. Nurs Stand 2011;26(5):48–56.
8. Irwin RS. Assessing cough severity and efficacy of therapy in clinical research: ACCP evidence-based clinical practice guidelines. Chest 2006;129(Suppl 1): 222S–31S.
9. Crapo RO, Casaburi R, Coates AL, et al. Guidelines for methacholine and exercise challenge testing-1999. Am J Respir Crit Care Med 2000;161(1):309–29.
10. Miller MR, Hankinson J, Brusasco V, et al, ATS/ERS Task Force. Standardisation of spirometry. Eur Respir J 2005;26:319–38.
11. Busse W. Asthma diagnosis and treatment: filling in the information gaps. J Allergy Clin Immunol 2011;128:740–9.
12. Anderson SD, Charlton B, Weiler JM, et al. Comparison of mannitol and methacholine to predict exercise-induced bronchoconstriction and a clinical diagnosis of asthma. Respir Res 2009;10:4.
13. McCormack M, Enright PL. Making the diagnosis of asthma. Respir Care 2008; 53(5):583–92.
14. Dweik RA, Boggs PB, Erzurum SC, et al. An official ATS clinical practice guideline: interpretation of exhaled nitric oxide levels (FeNO) for clinical applications. Am J Respir Crit Care Med 2011;184:602–15.
15. Majid H, Kao C. Utility of exhaled nitric oxide in the diagnosis and management of asthma. Curr Opin Pulm Med 2010;16:42–7.

Asthma in Primary Care
A Case-based Review of Pharmacotherapy

Raechel Ferry-Rooney, MSN, APRN-ANP[a,b],*

KEYWORDS

- Asthma • Primary care • Bronchodilators • Inhaled steroids • Primary care providers
- Asthma control

KEY POINTS

- Primary care providers work in partnership with the patient for effective asthma management. The Primary care provider is in a unique position of knowing the patient and the patient's financial and personal circumstances to help determine a treatment that is the most appropriate fit for the patient's individual circumstances.
- Asthma can be a costly disease. Patients often find it financially challenging. Half of the uninsured individuals with asthma cannot afford their prescription medications, and approximately 1 in 9 insured people cannot afford their prescription medications.
- Recurrent history of wheezing, cough (especially at night), shortness of breath, and chest tightness is highly suggestive of asthma.
- Many inhaler devices are now dry powder and breath activated. If the device is a meter dose inhaler and not breath activated, the best technique for use is to add a spacer device. The spacer device assists in proper medication delivery. Proper medication delivery is important because up to 70% of patients do not use the multidose inhaler correctly. When the inhaler is placed directly into the mouth and the canister is depressed, it is difficult to coordinate the timing of inhalation with medication release and often the patient does not receive the intended dose of medication into the lungs.
- Inhaled corticosteroids remain the cornerstone in treatment of symptom-persistent asthma. They serve an important function in treating the underlying inflammation seen in patients with persistent asthma.

OVERVIEW

Asthma is a disease of increasing prevalence and cost within the United States and worldwide. Asthma prevalence in the United States increased from 7.3% in 2001 to 8.4% in 2010, when 25.7 million persons had asthma.[1] Prevalence was higher among

No disclosures to report.
a Adult and Gerontology Nurse Practitioner Program, College of Nursing, Rush University, 600 South Paulina Street, Chicago, IL 60612, USA; b Department of Internal Medicine, University of Illinois Medical Center, 1801 W Taylor St, Chicago, IL 60612, USA
* College of Nursing, Rush University, 600 South Paulina Street, Chicago, IL 60612.
E-mail address: raechel_ferry_rooney@rush.edu

http://dx.doi.org/10.1016/j.cnur.2012.12.005
0029-6465/13/$ – see front matter © 2013 Elsevier Inc. All rights reserved.

children than in adults, and higher among people of color than persons of European descent.[1] It is estimated that asthma is responsible for about 15 million annual outpatient visits to health care providers and for nearly 2 million annual inpatient hospital days of treatment.[2]

Asthma remains the 14th leading diagnosis for ambulatory care settings, with half of all visits being within the primary care office.[3] According to the Centers of Disease Control and Prevention, primary care settings continue to be the site of opportunity for effective asthma management, promoting better management and a decrease in emergency room visits.[4] The cost of asthma both to the patient and to the nation in loss of productivity continues to be an area of concern. Asthma costs in the United States grew from about $53 billion in 2002 to about $56 billion, a 6% increase, in 2007.[5]

Prescription medications along with office visits represented most asthma expenses.[6] Currently 1 in 2 uninsured individuals with asthma cannot afford their prescription medications, and approximately 1 in 9 insured people cannot afford their prescription medications.[5]

In reviewing these statistics, it is clear that asthma is a leading cause of illness and financial burden for those with the disease. As noted by the Centers of Disease Control and Prevention, primary care providers (PCP) are the ideal providers to work in partnership with the patient to identify and control asthma symptoms. The PCP is in a unique position of knowing the patient and the patient's financial and personal circumstances to best determine a treatment that is the most appropriate fit for the patient's life. According to the Institutes of Medicine, primary care is "the provision of integrated, accessible health care services by clinicians who are accountable for addressing a large majority of personal health care needs, developing a sustained partnership with patients, and practicing in the context of family and community."[7]

CASE

Rhonda is a 31-year-old woman who presents to the office as a new patient. She has been seen infrequently and inconsistently by primary care because she is a working parent with 3 children aged 4 to 15 years. She states she is motivated to come to see you today because of a 2-year history of a cough. Her cough is varied, occurring often at night, at minimum 3 times weekly. It can be hacking to the point of vomiting. She rarely coughs up sputum but notes she feels it in her throat. She does notice occasional wheezing, especially with unexpected exercise, like running for a bus. She admits to shortness of breath especially with exercise, but also admits she attributes it to her weight. She denies fever, weight loss, and night sweats.

On further discussion, Rhonda has had a diagnosis of asthma since she was pregnant with her oldest child 15 years ago. Since that time, she has been prescribed or has borrowed albuterol inhalers periodically when she feels that her wheezing is bad. She has had urgent care for her asthma about 4 times since she was diagnosed. She has been to an emergency department once with wheezing and was treated and released. She notes that a few times she has been given "that purple" inhaler when she has been seen in a clinic. Currently she has been out of any inhaler for 4 months.

Rhonda's past medical history is significant for seasonal allergy and allergy to dust and cats. She does not take any medications for this currently. She has no allergies to medications or foods of which she is aware. She denies any additional medical history. She is not taking any medications of her own currently. She will use her son's albuterol inhaler if she needs it. She takes no other medications.

Her family history is significant for a son with asthma and allergies. He is also on "that purple" inhaler. Her brother had asthma as a child, but she states he "grew out of it." Rhonda does not smoke; she drinks alcohol twice monthly with friends, usually vodka-mixed drinks. She denies any illicit drug use and no herbals or supplements. She lives in a rental apartment and does not live with any pets. Her current job is as a parking enforcement officer, so she is outdoors during her work shifts.

On examination, Rhonda is 5 ft 3 in and weighs 190 lb. Her body mass index is 33. Her blood pressure is controlled and she is afebrile. She is speaking easily with no distress noted. She is not currently coughing. You examine her head and note retracted tympanic membranes bilaterally, minimal injected conjunctiva bilaterally. Her nares are erythematous and swollen bilaterally with clear drainage, and no nasal polyps are noted. Her throat is injected with cobblestone appearance. Her tonsils are negative. Her chest reveals scattered end expiratory wheezes and no crackles. Her cardiac examination is unremarkable. Her skin reveals no eczema and no rashes.

The remainder of the examination is noncontributory.

You request a peak flow, which is 320 L/min. For her gender, age, and height, she should be able to blow about 430 L/min.[8] Rhonda is at 74% of expected. You order the administration of albuterol 4 puffs with spacer and instructions in a multidose inhaler (MDI) and spacer use with a recheck of the peak flow 1 hour after medication. The recheck is 390 L/min or 91% of expected with a 17% change after short-acting bronchodilators (SABAs), demonstrating a response to treatment.

The assessment of Rhonda is moderate persistent asthma that is currently active. A second assessment is allergic rhinosinusitis, which may be in part responsible for her worsened control. It is explained to her that her cough is a symptom of her asthma, and that by treating her allergies as well as her lungs, she will have better control of her asthma. An inhaled steroid is prescribed, to be used twice daily. It is stressed to use it regularly, not as needed. A SABA is also given, to be used every 4 hours as needed for wheeze, cough, or shortness of breath. Both inhalers should be used with a spacer device. Rhonda is provided instructions on medication and spacer use. It is explained to Rhonda that the spacer device will help the medication to reach her lung tissue rather than landing in her mouth. Last, a nasal steroid is prescribed to control her allergic rhinosinusitis.

As her provider, the advanced practice nurse (APN) considers providing Rhonda with a written asthma action plan, in that her symptoms are a part of her asthma. You instead give her written information containing medication use, step-up and step-down therapy, as well as the clinic's urgent phone contact information with instructions that, if she has any worsening symptoms or questions, she should call right away. You explain to her that this should serve as her asthma action plan until her next visit. You provide her with a brief explanation of her asthma action plan. She repeats back her daily medication, the dose and frequency, and explains back what medications she will take for her asthma symptoms as defined in her action plan. You tell her to call if the prescriptions are too expensive so that you can assist her in obtaining more affordable medications.[9] You will spend time with her on her asthma action plan on her next visit, which you schedule for 1 to 2 weeks.

CASE DISCUSSION

Rhonda's case is a very common scenario in the primary care setting. She has active asthma, which she has been treated for on many different occasions. She was not regularly followed by a provider and she has been lacking in education about her disease, its symptoms, and how to treat them. From her history you guess that "the purple inhaler" was likely a combination therapy of fluticasone and salmeterol.

She used it for a while, until it ran out, and no refill was obtained. This scenario recurred but she was lost to follow-up.

One of the most crucial considerations in patients such as Rhonda is patient/provider rapport.[10] The APN speaks to Rhonda in lay terms that she understands and with an approach that tells her it matters that she should feel better. She demonstrated during your conversation that she understood what she was being told. The APN feels confident that Rhonda will be back for her next appointment with less cough and more ability to live her busy life.

WHY A DIAGNOSIS OF ASTHMA?

According to the National Asthma Education and Prevention program (NAEPP),[11] the recurrent history of wheezing, cough (especially at night), shortness of breath, and chest tightness are highly suggestive of asthma. Rhonda reported cough for 2 years, which she especially noticed at night, and shortness of breath, especially with exercise. NAEPP states that symptoms that occur or worsen with exercise, viral infection, and irritants, among others, support a diagnosis of asthma.[11] In addition, the Global Initiative for Asthma[10] adds that when symptoms recur in a seasonal pattern or worsen around common allergens and irritants (**Box 1**), the suspicion for asthma increases. These facts in addition to Rhonda's history of a diagnosis of asthma and relief with inhaled steroids and albuterol confirm your diagnosis of asthma.

When approaching a patient with symptoms consistent with asthma, the provider must consider the other possible differential diagnoses of wheeze and cough. Some of these are listed in **Box 2**.

In many primary care offices there is no ready access to spirometry nor staff trained to perform the test. The peak flow meter is instead used, as in Rhonda's case. Although the Global Initiative for Asthma guidelines provide a role for peak flow monitoring as diagnostic, the NAEPP recommends spirometry to diagnose asthma. Peak flow is intended to monitor activity of the asthma and response to treatment.[10,11] Peak flow monitoring is most useful if compared with the patient's own previous

---

Box 1
Common allergens and irritants leading to asthma symptom occurrence

Animals with fur

Aerosol chemicals

Changes in temperature

Dust mites

Drugs: aspirin, β-blockers

Exercise

Pollen

Viral respiratory infections

Smoke

Strong emotional expression

Data from GINA: the Global Initiative for Asthma. Global strategy for asthma management and prevention. 2008. (updated 2011). Available at: http://www.ginasthma.com/Guidelineitem. asp??l1=2&l2=1&intId=1561; and Tarlo SM, Balmes J, Balkissoon R, et al. Diagnosis and management of work related asthma: American College of Chest Physicians Consensus Statement. Chest 2008;134:1S–41S.

Box 2
Differential diagnosis of asthma like symptoms in adults

- Chronic obstructive pulmonary disease
- Congestive heart failure
- Pulmonary embolism
- Mechanical obstruction of the airways (benign and malignant tumors)
- Pulmonary infiltration with eosinophilia
- Cough secondary to medications (ACE inhibitors)
- Vocal cord dysfunction

Data from National Asthma Education and Prevention Program. Expert panel report 3: guidelines for the diagnosis and management of asthma. Bethesda (MD): National Heart, Lung, and Blood Institute; 2007. Available at: http://www.nhlbi.nih.gov/guidelines/asthma/asthgdln.pdf.

---

readings. Less than 80% of the patient's normal best is considered abnormal and requires intervention.

Spirometry or pulmonary function testing can be ordered at a subsequent visit and periodically thereafter if the diagnosis remains unclear or if the patient does not respond to treatment as expected.

THE GOAL

What is our goal in our treatment of Rhonda?

- She should have symptom control such that she experiences as few symptoms of asthma as possible both day and night.
- Symptoms when experienced should be easily controlled with quick relief medications or step-up treatment.
- Understand her disease so that she can initiate her step-up treatment using her asthma action plan at home and call the PCP to be seen when needed.
- Importantly, she should not have any serious asthma exacerbations.
- She should have near normal lung function.[10]

TREATMENT OF ASTHMA

When approaching a patient such as Rhonda, the goal of the PCP should be to control her symptoms with the least medications possible while keeping the goals of treatment in mind. To achieve this, a determination of asthma severity is needed. In addition, the patient will need to be assessed for risk and impairment, which is determined by asthma symptoms as well as periodic spirometry. Rhonda's level of severity as previously discussed is moderately persistent, and her level of control is uncontrolled. Her risk by history is moderate because she has been to urgent care due to wheeze and breathlessness but has never been admitted to the hospital or intubated due to asthma.[11]

When discussing the possible choices of treatments for asthma patients, there are 2 classes to consider: quick relief medications and controller medications.

QUICK RELIEF MEDICATIONS

The mainstay of quick relief medications is SABAs. This category includes albuterol, levalbuterol, and pirbuterol. SABAs relax smooth muscle and are the treatment of choice for acute symptoms of wheezing, chest tightness, and cough.[11] Both albuterol and levalbuterol are dispensed via a MDI, which should be used with a spacer chamber for optimal efficacy. These medications are also available in a liquid form to be used in a nebulizer, should the patient be unable to use an MDI.

The adverse effects of the SABAs are important to note because they are common and can be disruptive. Many users will note tachycardia, tremor, anxiety, or irritation shortly after the use of SABAs. It is important to warn users to rinse out the mouth after use to decrease this occurrence. If patients find these symptoms especially difficult, or if anxiety is a comorbidity, the prescriber could consider levalbuterol, which may have less of these symptoms than the others. The current literature is yet unclear on this.

A second quick relief choice is the anticholinergics—ipratropium and tiotropium. Ipratropium inhibits muscarinic cholinergic receptors and reduces tone of the airway. Ipratropium is generally not recommended in place of SABAs, but rather in addition, especially in the acute care setting. There is very little comparison in the literature of SABAs and ipratropium in asthma.[8,10] More recently tiotropium has been studied for use in poorly controlled severe asthmatics for improvement in lung function. It can be added to inhaled corticosteroids (ICS) and long-acting β-agonist (LABA) for additional control.[12]

CONTROLLER MEDICATIONS

Although the choices for SABAs are few, the options for controller medications are vaster. The cornerstone of controller therapy for asthma is the inhaled corticosteroid.

Inhaled Corticosteroids

ICS are topical anti-inflammatory medications that reduce airway hyperresponsiveness and inhibit inflammatory cell migration and activation as well as block late phase reaction to allergens.[11] When used regularly, they reduce the hyperreactivity of the airway, achieving less airway restriction and better lung function. The user has fewer wheezing and coughing episodes and needs less SABA.

Many ICS are dispensed via an MDI, via a dry powder inhaler (DPI), or in a liquid formulation for use in a nebulizer. MDIs, as noted, require the use of a spacer chamber. DPIs are breath-activated devices and do not require the use of a spacer device. These devices do not require a spacer as the inhalation action dispenses the medication. A common side effect of ICS by MDI or DPI is thrush. The impact of this can be reduced by ensuring the patient rinse after inhalation. Rinsing is also recommended to reduce systemic absorption of ICS.

With the use of ICS, there is a minimal systemic absorption of the corticosteroid. In lower doses, systemic absorption is of minimal concern. However, with higher doses (750–850 µg), there can be hypothalamic-pituitary-adrenal suppression. In children, this can retard growth, as well as cause osteoporosis, glaucoma, cataracts, dermal thinning, and periodontal disease throughout the lifespan.[13]

Oral Steroids

Oral steroids are an important topic to mention as well. Oral steroids work systemically in the same way as ICS, but are more potent, working more quickly, especially in the setting of an acute exacerbation of asthma. A short burst of oral steroids is crucial in this setting, will usually result in a quick resolution of the exacerbation, and has few adverse effects. A recent study showed a direct correlation between time to first dose of oral steroid as directly impacting need to hospitalize acute asthma.[14] Years back, it was common to see long extended tapering of oral steroids in asthma. There is no evidence to show that a taper is necessary in short bursts (up to 10 days).[15] Patients should always be advised to take oral steroids with food to decrease the incidence of gastrointestinal (GI) upset or irritation and the potential for GI bleed, especially in those with a history of gastritis or previous GI bleeding.

Long-Acting Bronchodilators

LABAs were first marketed in the United States in 1990 as salmeterol. LABAs have greatly improved the breathlessness of symptom-persistent asthma since that time. There are 2 LABAs currently available—Salmeterol and formoterol. LABAs are recognized as a useful adjunct medication to ICS and SABAs. ICS and LABAs are available as combination therapy combined into 1 device. Two formulas are currently available as combination therapy. They are salmeterol and fluticasone or budesonide and formoterol. In 2005 the US Food and Drug Administration issued a black box warning alerting prescribers and the public to an increased risk of severe asthma exacerbations and asthma-related death when used without the concurrent use of an ICS. The effect was more pronounced in those of African American race than others. Since that time, the combination of ICS with LABA in 1 device has reduced this effect and is an appreciated second-line medication for those with asthma for whom ICS alone does not control breathlessness adequately.[16] LABAs have an up to 12-hour duration of bronchodilation and greatly add to the symptom control of persistent asthma.

Cromolyn Sodium and Nedocromil

Cromolyn sodium and nedocromil stabilize mast cells and interfere with chloride channel function. These medications have been off the market in the United States since 2010.

Immunomodulators

Immunomodulators are a recent addition to the treatment of severe persistent asthmatics with concurrent allergy to perennial allergens such as dust mite or cockroach. Omalizumab is a monoclonal antibody that prevents binding of immunoglobulin E (IgE) to receptors on basophils and mast cells.[11] It decreases free IgE levels rapidly and the expression of the high-affinity IgE receptor expression on key effector cells, including mast cells, basophils, dendritic cells, and monocytes.[17] Omalizumab should be reserved for severe persistent asthma only. It is very expensive and given by injection only. Importantly, there have been reports of anaphylaxis to omalizumab, and therefore, should only be performed in a clinical setting where emergency treatment is available.

Leukotriene Modifiers

Leukotriene modifiers interfere with the pathway of leukotriene mediators, which are released from mast cells, eosinophils, and basophils. They have been shown to have a positive effect on allergic rhinosinusitis as well as in mild persistent asthma.[11] It has been proposed that leukotriene modifiers have a more prominent role in the treatment of asthma. However, studies have not shown that these medications add to the symptom control of moderate or higher levels of asthma severity.[18] A meta-analysis performed in China showed that in mild to moderate asthma, adding leukotriene modifiers had a small but significant benefit to monotherapy with ICS alone. The studies did not show better control for severe asthma.[19]

Methylxanthines (Theophylline)

Methylxanthines (theophylline) are a mild to moderate oral bronchodilator that can be used as an alternative to LABAs. It may have mild anti-inflammatory effects. Methylxanthines are not preferred to other controller medications because there is wide inter-patient variability in the serum concentrations, and a narrow therapeutic index. It can have life-threatening toxicity and has been linked to cardiac arrhythmia and seizure.[15]

FUTURE MEDICATIONS

Most of the advancements in the asthma therapeutics are targeted toward the refractory severe persistent asthma. There have been little advancement for those with mild asthma.

With the aforementioned safety concerns with LABAs, scientists have looked at tiotropium, a long-acting anticholinergic typically used in chronic obstructive pulmonary disease for control of breathlessness and an increase in peak flows in severe persistent asthmatics. Results showed that tiotropium is equivalent to LABAs when used with ICS in this population. Tiotropium was not shown to be superior.[20] When tiotropium was added to ICS/LABA therapy, there was a significant increase in peak flows and no significant additional adverse effects on asthma health status or symptoms.[20]

There are multiple novel LABAs and long-acting antimuscarinics under development for use in at least moderate persistent asthmatics. Data are still pending regarding improvements in symptom control with the new agents.[20]

Much interest in attempting to target asthma treatment based on individual causation for those with moderate and severe symptoms exists, and studies have been promising. However preclinical use of various biologics targeting IgE and specific interleukins for prevention of the asthma response has been disappointing to date. Quirce and colleagues[20] state that future goals of treatment for this moderate to severe asthma population should be geared toward the expected asthma phenotype to individualize therapy.

A WORD ABOUT INHALER TECHNIQUE

It is imperative that patients be shown and given a return demonstration of how to use their MDI. Unless the delivery device is breath activated, an inhaler should be used with a spacer device. The spacer device assists the patient with timing of inhalation to medication actuation by holding the medication suspended in the spacer for subsequent inhalation into the lungs. This spacer device is important because up to 70% of patients do not use the MDI correctly.[21] When the inhaler is placed directly into the mouth and the canister is depressed, it is difficult to inhale quickly enough to receive the intended dose of medication into the lungs.[10,13,21,22]

FOLLOWING UP ON RHONDA

Rhonda returns for a follow-up visit in 1 week. She states she is feeling much better. She is using the inhaled steroid and the nasal steroid as prescribed. She complains that the co-pays on the medications were too high to also purchase the spacer device, so the pharmacist taught her appropriate MDI use without a spacer device. She says it was hard to do at first, but now she says she is "good at it." Rhonda states that she is not coughing now.

On examination, Rhonda's peak flow has increased to 400, which the APN now labels as her personal best. The APN explains this number may increase further, but that right now it is the best she has had. Her lungs are now free of wheeze. Her remaining examination is unremarkable.

The APN requests that Rhonda demonstrate her inhaler technique. On demonstration, her technique is not optimal. She is encouraged to consider purchasing a spacer device, explaining that this is a one-time expense. It is explained that she will feel even better when she is inhaling all of her medications.

Rhonda's tailored asthma action plan with her current personal best of 400 inserted is now further explained to her. She is provided a prescription for the oral steroid prednisone to be used if needed with the asthma action plan. A baseline spirometry test is scheduled now that Rhonda is feeling better. Rhonda is scheduled to return to the clinic in 6 weeks for a follow-up visit, or sooner if needed.

SUMMARY

Asthma remains a significant health burden on the population. PCPs are in an ideal position to be able to target treatment on an individual basis for patients in their care. It is important to determine the level of severity and control, evaluate the risk and impairment of the asthma patient, and then base the treatment on both the severity and the symptoms of disease. Additional consideration must be given to the patient's ability to be adherent to the therapy regimen.

ACKNOWLEDGMENTS

The author wishes to thank graduate student Kelly Grant, BSN, RN for her assistance in researching and reviewing this article.

REFERENCES

1. Akinabami L, Moorman J, Bailey C, et al. Trends in asthma prevalence, health-care use, and mortality in the United States, 2001-2010. NCHS Data Brief, 94. 2012. Available at: http://www.cdc.gov/nchs/data/databriefs/db94.htm.
2. Goldman L, Ausiello D. Cecil medicine. 24th edition. Philadelphia: Saunders/Elsevier; 2012.
3. Schappert S, Rechtsteiner E. Ambulatory medical care utilization estimates for 2007. Vital Health Stat 13 2011;(169). National Center for Health Statistics. Available at: http://www.cdc.gov/nchs/data/series/sr_13/sr13_169.pdf.
4. Centers for Disease Control and Prevention. QuickStats: health-care visits for asthma, by medical setting and health-insurance status — United States, 2003. MMWR Weekly 2006;54(14):405. Available at: http://www.cdc.gov/mmwr/preview/mmwrhtml/mm5514a8.htm.
5. Centers for Disease Control and Prevention. Asthma in the U.S. CDC Vital Signs. 2011. Available at: http://www.cdc.gov/vitalsigns/asthma.
6. Kamble S, Bharmal M. Incremental direct expenditure of treating asthma in the United States. J Asthma 2009;46(1):73–80. Available at: www.ncbi.nlm.nih.gov/pubmed/19191142.
7. Institute of Medicine of the National Academies. Primary care: American's health in a new era. Washington, DC: National Academy Press; 1996. p. 29.
8. Nunn AJ, Gregg I. New regression equations for predicting peak expiratory flow in adults. BMJ 1989;298(6680):1068–70.
9. Hodder R, Lougheed MD, Rowe BH, et al. Management of acute asthma in adults in the emergency department: nonventilatory management. CMAJ 2010;182(2): 55–67.

10. GINA: the Global Initiative for Asthma. Global strategy for asthma management and prevention. 2008. (updated 2011). Available at: http://guideline.gov/content.aspx?id=37283.

11. National Asthma Education and Prevention Program. Expert panel report 3: guidelines for the diagnosis and management of asthma. Bethesda (MD): National Heart, Lung, and Blood Institute; 2007. Available at: http://www.nhlbi.nih.gov/guidelines/asthma/asthgdln.pdf.

12. Kerstjens HA, Engel M, Dahl R, et al. Tiotropium in asthma poorly controlled with standard combination therapy. N Engl J Med 2012;367:1198–207.

13. Goroll AH, Mulley AG. Primary care medicine- office evaluation and management of the adult patient. 6th edition. Philadelphia: Lippincott Williams and Wilkins; 2009.

14. Lougheed MD, Garvey N, Chapman KR, et al. Variations and gaps in management of acute asthma in ontario emergency departments. Chest 2009;135:724–36.

15. Chisholm-Burns MA, Schwinghammer TL, Wells BG, et al. Pharmacotherapy principles and practice. 2nd edition. New York: McGraw Hill; 2010.

16. Dahl R, Chuchalin A, Gor D, et al. EXCEL: a randomised trial comparing salmeterol/fluticasone propionate and fomotorol/budensonide combinations in adults with persistent asthma. Respir Med 2006;100:1152–62.

17. Dimov W, Casale TB. Immunomodulators for Asthma. Allergy Asthma Immunol Res 2010;2(4):228–34.

18. Katial RK, Oppenheimer JJ, Ostrom NK, et al. Adding Montelukast to Fluticasone Propionate/salmeterol for control of asthma and seasonal allergic rhinitis. Allergy Asthma Proc 2010;31:68–75.

19. Cao Y, Wang J, Bunjhoo H, et al. Comparison of leukotriene receptor antagonists in addition to inhaled corticosteroid and inhaled corticosteroid alone in the treatment of adolescents and adults with bronchial asthma: a meta-analysis. Asian Pac J Allergy Immunol 2012;30(2):130–8. Available at: http://www.nejm.org/doi/full/10.1056/NEJMe1108666?viewType=Print.

20. Quirce S, Bobolea I, Baranco P. Emerging drugs for asthma. Expert Opin Emerg Drugs 2012;17(2):219–37.

21. Dolovich MB, Eng P, Ahrens RC, et al. Device selection and outcomes of aerosol therapy: evidence-based guidelines. Chest 2005;127:335–71. Available at: www.chestjournal.org. Accessed January 19, 2007.

22. Lareau SC, Hodder R. Teaching inhaler use in chronic obstructive pulmonary disease patients. J Am Acad Nurse Pract 2012;24(2):113–20.

A Guideline-based Approach to Asthma Management

Catherine "Casey" S. Jones, PhD, RN, ANP-C, AE-C[a,*],
Ellen A. Becker, PhD, RRT-NPS, RPFT, AE-C[b],
Catherine D. Catrambone, PhD, RN[c], Molly A. Martin, MD, MAPP[d]

KEYWORDS

- Asthma • Asthma guidelines • Asthma severity • Asthma control
- Guideline adherence

KEY POINTS

- Clinical guidelines are available for the diagnosis and management of asthma.
- Asthma assessment includes an evaluation of asthma severity and asthma control.
- Asthma severity and control include assessments of impairment and risk.
- Strategies to improve guideline adherence should include a multidimensional system-based approach.

INTRODUCTION

Despite an increased understanding of asthma mechanisms and improved treatment approaches, asthma prevalence and morbidity remain high both nationally[1] and internationally.[2] Clinical practice guidelines have evolved to disseminate best practice diagnosis and treatment recommendations to clinicians with the goal of improving asthma care and the quality of life for persons with asthma.[2,3] Guidelines have been available since 1992[4] and provide evidence to support their efficacy in improving outcomes for persons with asthma; however there remains a notable gap between guideline-recommended care and current care practices.[5–9] The failure to fully adopt and implement guidelines is partially attributed to providers. Physician adherence is affected by physician workflow and awareness of asthma guideline structure and content,[10] lack of outcome expectancy, and poor provider self-efficacy.[9] Communication, training and workload[11] and factors at the individual, organizational and

[a] Texas Pulmonary and Critical Care Consultants, PA, Texas Woman's University, Suite 403, 1604 Hospital Parkway, Bedford, TX 76022, USA; [b] Respiratory Care, Rush University College of Health Professions, 600 S. Paulina, 750 Armour Academic Center, Chicago, IL 60612, USA; [c] Adult Health and Gerontological Nursing, Rush University College of Nursing, 600 S. Paulina, 1064B Armour Academic Center, Chicago, IL 60612, USA; [d] Department of Preventive Medicine, Rush University Medical Center, 1700 W Van Buren, Suite 470, Chicago, IL 60612, USA
* Corresponding author.
E-mail address: cjones29@twu.edu

Nurs Clin N Am 48 (2013) 35–45
http://dx.doi.org/10.1016/j.cnur.2012.12.007
0029-6465/13/$ – see front matter © 2013 Elsevier Inc. All rights reserved.

environmental levels[12] were identified as barriers influencing nursing adherence to practice guidelines.

The National Asthma Education Prevention Program (NAEPP) of the National Heart, Lung, and Blood Institute (NHLBI) convened three Expert Panels to prepare the most recent guidelines for the diagnosis and management of asthma. The 2007 Expert Panel Report 3: *Guidelines for the Diagnosis and Management of Asthma* (EPR-3)[3] centers around four components of effective asthma management including asthma severity and control; environmental factors and comorbid conditions affecting asthma; education for patient/provider partnership in asthma care; and pharmacologic therapy. The purpose of this article is to provide an overview of the EPR-3 guidelines for asthma management. Emphasis will be on the assessment of asthma severity and control using a case-based approach and strategies to improve guideline adherence.

CASE STUDY

Ms Jenkins is a 27-year-old female who has been struggling with wheezing, cough and chest tightness intermittently for the last two months. She has not been exposed to anyone who has been ill. She notes that she has been waking up at night due to short-ness of breath for the last three nights, and that she has had difficulty climbing stairs at work for weeks. This last week she has been having symptoms on a daily basis. She was prescribed an albuterol inhaler last year due to an episode of "bronchitis" and has been using this inhaler twice a day for the last week.

The clinician's first task is to establish that Ms Jenkins has asthma, at which time the *severity* of her asthma will be determined. *Treatment* will then be initiated. Over time, *control* will be assessed and treatment modified. In the EPR-3 guidelines,[3] the concepts of severity and control guide the comprehensive assessment required for asthma management. The overall goals of asthma therapy are to reduce impairment and reduce risk. The EPR-3 guidelines contain specific tables that address severity, control, and the step-wise approach for managing asthma. These tools are classified according to age; youths ≥12 years of age to adults (**Figs. 1–3**), children 5–11 years of age, and children 0–4 years of age.

Spirometry is performed in the clinician's office and the results are provided in **Table 1**. The pre-bronchodilator spirometry results suggest moderate obstruction, while post-bronchodilator spirometry normalized after two puffs of albuterol, a short-acting β_2-agonist (SABA). Her FEV_1 increased 26% after using albuterol. To make a diagnosis of asthma, we must demonstrate both a 12% increase in FEV_1 and 200 mL increase in FEV_1. Ms Jenkins' spirometry results reveal that she has achieved both criteria and therefore has asthma.

SEVERITY

Severity refers to the intrinsic characteristics of asthma for an individual. Asthma severity is subdivided into intermittent or persistent, and persistent disease is further divided into mild, moderate, or severe persistent. The EPR-3 guidelines recommend that initial medical management for patients taking no inhaled corticosteroid medications be based upon the patient's severity classification. In Ms Jenkins' case, she has daily symptoms, she uses albuterol twice a day for symptom relief, she has difficulty climbing stairs at work, and an FEV_1 pre-bronchodilator spirometry value that was 65% predicted. This categorizes her severity as moderate persistent (see **Fig. 1**). She also has been waking up at night due to asthma symptoms for three nights in the past month which is consistent with mild persistent asthma. When symptoms and test results fall into more than one category, as with Ms Jenkins, the highest

Classification of Asthma Severity (≥12 years of age)

Components of Severity		Intermittent	Persistent Mild	Persistent Moderate	Persistent Severe
Impairment Normal FEV$_1$/FVC: 8-19 yr 85% 20-39 yr 80% 40-59 yr 75% 60-80 yr 70%	Symptoms	≤2 days/week	>2 days/week but not daily	Daily	Throughout the day
	Nighttime awakenings	≤2x/month	3-4x/month	>1x/week but not nightly	Often 7x/week
	Short-acting beta$_2$-agonist use for symptom control (not prevention of EIB)	≤2 days/week	>2 days/week but not daily, and not more than 1x on any day	Daily	Several times per day
	Interference with normal activity	None	Minor limitation	Some limitation	Extremely limited
	Lung function	•Normal FEV$_1$ between exacerbations •FEV$_1$ >80% predicted •FEV$_1$/FVC normal	•FEV$_1$ >80% predicted •FEV$_1$/FVC normal	•FEV$_1$ >60% but <80% predicted •FEV$_1$/FVC reduced 5%	•FEV$_1$ <60% predicted •FEV$_1$/FVC reduced >5%
Risk	Exacerbations requiring oral systemic corticosteroids	0-1/year (see note)	≥ 2/year(see note)		
		Consider severity and interval since last exacerbation. Frequency and severity may fluctuate over time for patients in any severity category Relative annual risk of exacerbations may be related to FEV$_1$			
Recommended Step for Initiating Treatment		Step 1	Step 2	Step 3 and consider short course of oral systemic corticosteroids	Step 4 or 5
		In 2-6 weeks, evaluate level of asthma control that is achieved and adjust therapy accordingly			

Fig. 1. Classifying asthma severity and initiating treatment in youths ≥12 years of age and adults. Assessing severity and initiating treatment for patients who are not currently taking long-term control medications. The stepwise approach is meant to assist, not replace the clinical decision-making required to meet individual patient needs. Level of severity is determined by assessment of both impairment and risk. Assess impairment domain by patient's/caregiver's recall of previous 2–4 weeks and spirometry. Assign severity to the most severe category in which any feature occurs. At present, there are inadequate data to correspond frequencies of exacerbations with different levels of asthma severity. In general, more frequent and intense exacerbations (eg, requiring urgent, unscheduled care, hospitalization, or ICU admission) indicate greater underlying disease severity. For treatment purposes, patients who had ≥2 exacerbations requiring oral systemic corticosteroids in the past year may be considered the same as patients who have persistent asthma, even in the absence of impairment levels consistent with persistent asthma.[3]

Components of Control		Classification of Asthma Control (≥12 years of age)		
		Well Controlled	Not Well Controlled	Very Poorly Controlled
Impairment	Symptoms	≤2 days/week	>2 days/week	Throughout the day
	Nighttime awakenings	≤2x/month	1-3x/week	≥4x/week
	Interference with normal activity	None	Some limitation	Extremely limited
	Short-acting beta$_2$-agonist use for symptom control (not prevention of EIB)	≤2 days/week	>2 days/week	Several times per day
	FEV$_1$ or peak flow	>80% predicted/personal best	60-80% predicted/personal best	<60% predicted/personal best
	Validated Questionnaires ATAQ ACQ ACT	0 ≤0.75* ≥20	1-2 ≥1.5 16-19	3-4 N/A ≤15
Risk	Exacerbations requiring oral systemic corticosteroids	0-1/year	≥2/year (see note)	
			Consider severity and interval since last exacerbation	
	Progressive loss of lung function	Evaluation requires long-term follow-up care.		
	Treatment-related adverse effects	Medication side effects can vary in intensity from none to very troublesome and worrisome. The level of intensity does not correlate to specific levels of control but should be considered in the overall assessment of risk.		
Recommended Action for Treatment		•Maintain current step. •Regular follow ups every 1-6 months to maintain control. •Consider step down if well controlled for at least 3 months.	•Step up 1 step and •Reevaluate in 2-6 weeks. •For side effects, consider alternative treatment options.	•Consider short course of oral systemic corticosteroids, •Step up 1-2 steps, and •Reevaluate in 2 weeks. •For side effects, consider alternative treatment options.

severity criterion is used. Therefore, we will categorize her asthma as moderate persistent. The asthma symptoms, nighttime awakenings, albuterol use, interference with normal activity and lung function constitute the *impairment* domain of asthma severity. While severity classification can sometimes be challenging,[13] it is an important step before developing a treatment plan.

A second domain of severity is the determination of *risk*. Risk is the potential for adverse events in the future including exacerbations, and progressive, irreversible loss of pulmonary function. A greater risk exists for patients who have required hospital admissions, intensive care unit stays, and frequent emergency department visits. Further, patients with low impairment might be at high risk for severe, even life-threatening asthma exacerbations.[14] Patients may also incur future risks from progressive loss of lung function.[3] Risk is present at every level of severity and an evaluation of the patient's risk for negative outcomes is important to assess at every visit. While Ms Jenkins' impairment domain criteria demonstrated a moderate persistent severity classification, her risk assessment is low because she had no prior exacerbations in the past year. Thus, her asthma severity remains classified as moderate persistent. If she had reported frequent exacerbations requiring oral corticosteroids, her risk would be high and we would consider elevating her severity classification to severe persistent.

Technically, we cannot classify severity in patients who are already using inhaled corticosteroid medications. These medications alter lung function and symptoms, thereby creating an inaccurate picture of intrinsic lung function. When this happens, a severity classification can be inferred from the lowest doses of medication required to control asthma symptoms.[3] Many clinicians inappropriately use the severity table with patients who are taking inhaled corticosteroid medications[15] rather than evaluate the lowest dose of medication needed to control asthma symptoms. For example, if Ms Jenkins were well controlled on a low-dose inhaled corticosteroid (ICS) plus long-acting beta$_2$-agonist (LABA) (Step 3), she would be classified as moderate persistent because Step 3 medications correlate with moderate severity (see **Fig. 1**).

Initial treatment of asthma is based upon the patient's severity classification.[3] The bottom section of the severity table (see **Fig. 1**) lists the corresponding step for starting therapy. Initial treatment for Ms Jenkins' moderate persistent asthma is Step 3. Using a stepwise approach, either a low-dose ICS plus LABA or a medium-dose ICS would be initiated (see **Fig. 3**). An alternative Step 3 therapy is also provided. The specific choice will be influenced by the dialogue that emerges from the partnership between the patient and provider. Ms Jenkins was started on a low-dose ICS and LABA to be

◄—————————————————————————————————————

Fig. 2. Assessing asthma control and adjusting therapy in youth ≥12 years of age and adults. The stepwise approach is meant to assist, not replace, the clinical decision making required to meet individual patient needs. The level of control is based on the most severe impairment or risk category. Assess impairment domain by patient's recall of previous 2–4 weeks and by spirometry/or peak flow measures. Symptom assessment for longer periods should reflect a global assessment, such as inquiring whether the patient's asthma is better or worse since the last visit. At present, there are inadequate data to correspond frequencies of exacerbations with different levels of asthma control. In general, more frequent and intense exacerbations (eg, requiring urgent, unscheduled care, hospitalization, or ICU admission) indicate poorer disease control. For treatment purposes, patients who had ≥2 exacerbations requiring oral systemic corticosteroids in the past year may be considered the same as patients who have not-well-controlled asthma, even in the absence of impairment levels consistent with not-well-controlled asthma.[3]

Persistent Asthma: Daily Medication

Consult with asthma specialist if step 4 care or higher is required. Consider consultation at step 3.

Intermittent Asthma

Step 1

Preferred:
SABA PRN

Step 2

Preferred:
Low-dose ICS

Alternative:
Cromolyn, LTRA, Nedocromil, or Theophylline

Step 3

Preferred:
Low dose ICS + LABA OR medium-dose ICS

Alternative:
low-dose ICS + either LTRA, Theophylline, or Zileuton

Step 4

Preferred:
Medium-dose ICS + LABA

Alternative:
Medium-dose ICS+either LTRA, Theophylline, or Zileuton

Step 5

Preferred:
High-dose ICS + LABA

AND

Consider Omalizumab for patients who have allergies

Step 6

Preferred:
High-dose ICS + LABA + oral corticosteroid

AND

Consider Omalizumab for patients who have allergies

Step up if needed
(first, check adherence, environmental control, and comorbid conditions)

Assess control

Step down if possible
(and asthma is well controlled at least 3 months)

Each step: Patient education, environmental control, and management of comorbidities.
Steps 2-4: Consider subcutaneous allergen immunotherapy for patients who have allergic asthma *

Quick-Relief Medication for All Patients

SABA as needed for symptoms. Intensity of treatment depends on severity of symptoms: up to 3 treatments at 20-minute intervals as needed. Short course of oral systemic corticosteroids may be needed

Caution: Increasing use of SABA or use >2 days a week for symptom relief (not prevention of EIB) generally indicates inadequate control and the need to step up treatment.

Table 1
Result of Ms Jenkins' spirometry in office

	Pre-Bronchodilator	Post-Bronchodilator

FVC % Predicted
FVC = forced vital capacity: The total
   volume of air exhaled during a forced
   exhalation after a full inspiration.
	82%	85%

FEV$_1$ % Predicted
FEV$_1$ = forced expiratory volume in
   1 second: The volume of air exhaled
   in 1 s during a forced exhalation after
   a full inspiration.
	65%	82%

FEV$_1$/FVC (%) FEV$_1$/FVC = The ratio of the individual's FEV$_1$/FVC.	66%	84%

taken daily with a SABA as needed. Asthma self-management education should also be initiated at this time and a written asthma action plan provided.[3] It is critical to explain to Ms Jenkins that she will not feel the same immediate relief from her ICS medication, but she will obtain relief from the LABA and SABA. It takes 4–8 weeks of regular use for the benefits of the ICS to be apparent. Routine use of an ICS needs to be emphasized, and teaching her proper technique with the new inhaler is essential. Patients need detailed instructions, practice, and sometimes assistive devices such as spacers for metered dose inhalers. Finally, it is critical to address potential barriers to medication adherence that Ms Jenkins may have such as an inability to pay for her medications or fears about routine use of an ICS medication.

CONTROL

Ms Jenkins returned to clinic 8 weeks later. She reported no episodes of wheezing, nighttime awakenings, or SABA use. She was able to regularly attend work. Her

◄───

Fig. 3. Stepwise approach for managing asthma in youths ≥12 years of age and adults. The stepwise approach is meant to assist, not replace, the clinical decision making required to meet individual patient needs. If alternative treatment is used and response is inadequate, discontinue it and use the preferred treatment before stepping up. Zileuton is a less desirable alternative because of limited studies as adjunctive therapy and the need to monitor liver function. Theophylline requires monitoring of serum concentration levels. In step 6, before oral systemic corticosteroids are introduced, a trial of high-dose ICS + inhaled long-acting beta$_2$ agonist (LABA) + leukotriene receptor agonist (LTRA), theophylline, or zileuton may be considered, although this approach has not been studied in clinical trials. Step 1, 2, and 3 preferred therapies are based on evidence A; step 3 alternative therapy is based on evidence A for LTRA, evidence B for theophylline, and evidence D for zileuton. Step 4 preferred therapy is based on evidence B, and alternative therapy is based on evidence B for LTRA and theophylline and evidence D for zileuton. Step 5 preferred therapy is based on evidence B. Step 6 preferred therapy is based on (EPR-2 1997) and evidence B for omalizumab. Immunotherapy for steps 2 to 4 is based on evidence B for house-dust mites, animal danders, and pollens; evidence is weak or lacking for molds and cockroaches. Evidence is strongest for immunotherapy with single allergens. The role of allergy in asthma is greater in children than in adults. Clinicians who administer immunotherapy should be prepared and equipped to identify and treat anaphylaxis that may occur.[3]

Asthma Control Test (ACT) score was 23 and FEV$_1$ was 82% predicted pre-bronchodilator. She reported taking her low-dose ICS and LABA regularly.

Once severity has been established and treatment initiated, we shift to the assessment of asthma control.[2,3] The three categories of control are well controlled, not well controlled, and very poorly controlled. An assessment of Ms Jenkins' symptoms, night-time awakenings, SABA use, FEV$_1$ and ACT score all fell within the well controlled classification for impairment (see **Fig. 2**). Her risk assessment showed that she did not require an oral corticosteroid for her exacerbation. Although Ms Jenkins' asthma is well controlled based upon her symptoms and her FEV$_1$, her treatment requires ongoing evaluation. How often does she use her SABA inhaler? Using the SABA inhaler for symptoms (other than routine exercise) more than twice a week indicates that her asthma would not be in good control. Fortunately, Ms Jenkins has not needed to use her SABA recently. Should Ms Jenkins' medication therapy be reduced? Stepping down medication therapy should be delayed until there is at least three months of good asthma control. If in the future she requires a step up in therapy, review her exposure to environmental triggers, medication adherence and inhaler technique, elements that should be monitored at each encounter. If control cannot be obtained, other factors like allergic rhinitis, gastroesophageal reflux disease (GERD), and vocal cord dysfunction should be considered.[3] The emphasis on monitoring asthma control is a departure from the Expert Panel Report 2 guidelines released in 1997[16] which contained a single assessment, severity, and used the severity assessment to guide asthma treatment.

In summary, good asthma management includes assessment of asthma control and severity. Asthma severity classification is used to characterize the intrinsic nature of the disease in an individual and to guide treatment recommendations. The EPR-3 guidelines tables can be used to categorize symptoms and test data into impairment and risk domains, ultimately yielding a severity category. The treatment recommendation tables then can be appropriately applied. Other guidelines take a similar approach with the exception that the Global Initiative for Asthma (GINA) includes two constructs for the severity measure; treatment intensity — the treatment needed to control a patient's asthma symptoms (the severity of the underlying disease) and responsiveness to therapy.[2] After severity has been established and treatment initiated, the EPR-3 guidelines should be used to assess asthma control on a regular basis. Control will guide decisions about the need to step up or step down therapy. Although less critical for routine asthma management decisions, asthma severity plays an important role for population-based evaluations, research studies, or reevaluation of the patient's disease.[15] The features of asthma control and severity are outlined in **Table 2**.

Several validated questionnaires have been developed to standardize the assessment of asthma control. The EPR-3 guidelines refer to several of these questionnaires which include the Asthma Control Test (ACT) for adults[17] and children,[18] Asthma Control Questionnaire ©[19] and the Asthma Therapy Assessment Questionnaire © (ATAQ).[20]

GUIDELINE IMPLEMENTATION

Guideline-based care cannot improve outcomes unless they are effectively implemented. Following the release of EPR-3 guidelines, the NAEPP convened a Guidelines Implementation Panel (GIP) that published a guide to provide practical applications for the use of guidelines in the field. *Partners Putting Practice into Action*[21] emphasizes six priority EPR-3 messages that include asthma severity and control and highlight the evidence-based recommendations. In addition to the three core themes of communication, systems integration and patient/provider support, the GIP provided strategies

Table 2
Asthma control and severity characteristics

Feature	Control	Severity
Definition	Degree to which manifestations of asthma are minimized and treatment goals are met	Intrinsic intensity of the patient's asthma GINA guidelines define severity as the intensity of treatment needed to treat patient's asthma symptoms (severity of underlying disease) and responsiveness to treatment[2]
Variability	Changes more frequently	More stable, but can change over time
Functions	Maintain or adjust therapy by step up or step down	Descriptive for population studies and research Reevaluation of the patient's condition over time
Assessment frequency	Every encounter	Initial diagnosis, new to provider, suspicion that characteristics of underlying disease have changed

Data from National Asthma Education and Prevention Program. Expert panel report 3 (EPR-3): Guidelines for the diagnosis and management of asthma - Full report 2007. NIH Publication Number 08-5846; 2007.

for dynamic engagement of stakeholders and a host of implementation approaches to promote guideline use. Eleven strategies were recommended that include (p 17):

- Gathering information with respect to message barriers/solutions for identified priority audiences
- Convene knowledge brokers, influential leaders and decision makers
- Pilot test strategies
- Provide professional education and training
- Provide point-of service prompting
- Conduct quality improvement
- Provide patient-self management education
- Promote financing support systems
- Strengthen linkages between medical and community-based resources
- Collate, analyze and share data
- Disseminate and market the National Asthma Control Initiatives (NACI) activities, results and products.

These strategies can help guide system-level changes in asthma care. For example, the electronic health record (EHR) provides an effective platform to implement point-of-service prompting to improve adherence with asthma guidelines. Nkoy and colleagues[22] implemented an asthma-specific reminder and decision support (RADS) system within the EHR that improved compliance with pediatric asthma inpatient quality measures. Kowk[23] found that use of an asthma clinical assessment form and electronic decision support system resulted in improved compliance with and documentation of asthma severity and discharge management plans in the emergency department. Bell and colleagues[24] used an asthma decision support system across several pediatric primary care practices and demonstrated an increased prescription rate for controller medications, greater spirometry use, updated asthma action plans.

Other approaches to assist in the integration of guidelines into clinical practice integrate multiple strategies. Boulet and colleagues[25] outlined steps for a GINA guideline implementation program that can be applied and adopted according to local conditions, as well as a broader context. Some of the elements in this model include identifying stakeholders, performing a needs assessment, identifying care gaps and key messages to convey; and developing and prioritizing implementation strategies, metrics, resources, and detailed implementation plans. Alvanzo and colleagues[26] reported that a combination of education, motivation, and facilitation fostered successful guideline implementation.

The EPR-3 guidelines provide a comprehensive framework for managing patients with asthma. These guidelines include an ongoing assessment of asthma control and severity, stepwise medication management, environmental control, and education for a partnership in care. To tackle the barriers limiting the widespread implementation of guideline-recommended care, a systems-based approach should be used.

REFERENCES

1. Moorman JE, Akinbami LJ, Bailey CM, et al. National surveillance of asthma: United States, 2001-2010. National Center for Health Statistics. Vital Health Stats 2012;35(3).
2. Global Initiative for Asthma. Global strategy for asthma management and prevention 2012 (update). 2012. p. 128.
3. National Asthma Education and Prevention Program, Third expert panel on the diagnosis and management of asthma. Expert panel report 3: guidelines for the diagnosis and management of asthma. NIH Publication No. 07-4051; 2007.
4. Fitzgerald ST. National Asthma Education Program Expert Panel report: guidelines for the diagnosis and management of asthma. AAOHN J 1992;40(8):376–82.
5. Murphy K, Meltzer E, Blaiss M, et al. Asthma management and control in the United States: results of the 2009 Asthma Insight and Management survey. Allergy Asthma Proc 2012;33(1):54–6.
6. Rance K, O'Laughlen M, Ting S. Improving asthma care for African American children by increasing national asthma guideline adherence. J Pediatr Health Care 2011;25(4):235–49.
7. Weinstein AG. The potential of asthma adherence management to enhance asthma guidelines. Ann Allergy Asthma Immunol 2011;106(4):283–91.
8. Navaratnam P, Jayawant SS, Pedersen CA, et al. Physician adherence to the national asthma prescribing guidelines: evidence from national outpatient survey data in the United States. Ann Allergy Asthma Immunol 2008;100(3):216.
9. Wisnivesky JP, Lorenzo J, Lyn-Cook R, et al. Barriers to adherence to asthma management guidelines among inner-city primary care providers. Ann Allergy Asthma Immunol 2008;101(3):264.
10. Bracha Y, Brottman G, Carlson A. Physicians, guidelines, and cognitive tasks. Eval Health Prof 2011;34(3):309–35.
11. Abrahamson K, Fox R, Doebbeling B. Facilitators and barriers to clinical practice guideline use among nurses. Am J Nurs 2012;112(7):26–35.
12. Ploeg J, Davies B, Edwards N, et al. Factors influencing best-practice guideline implementation: lessons learned from administrators, nursing staff, and project leaders. Worldviews Evid Based Nurs 2007;4(4):210–9.
13. Graham L. Classifying asthma. Chest 2006;130(1 Suppl):13S–20S.
14. Ayres J, Jyothish D, Ninan T. Brittle asthma. Paediatr Respir Rev 2004;5(1):40–4.
15. Taylor DR, Bateman ED, Boulet L, et al. A new perspective on concepts of asthma severity and control. Eur Respir J 2008;32(3):545–54.

16. National Institutes of Health. Practical guide for the diagnosis and management of asthma. Washington, DC: US Department of Health and Human Services, National Institutes of Health; 1997. Publication no. 97–4053.
17. Nathan RA, Sorkness CA, Kosinski M, et al. Development of the asthma control test: a survey for assessing asthma control. J Allergy Clin Immunol 2004;113(1): 59–65.
18. Liu AH, Zeiger R, Sorkness C, et al. Development and cross-sectional validation of the Childhood Asthma Control Test. J Allergy Clin Immunol 2007;119(4): 817–25.
19. Juniper E, Guyatt G, Ferrie P, et al. Development and validation of a questionnaire to measure asthma control. Eur Respir J 2001;14(4):902–7.
20. Vollmer WM, Markson LE, O'connor E, et al. Association of asthma control with health care utilization and quality of life. Am J Respir Crit Care Med 1999;160(5): 1647–52.
21. U.S. Department of Health and Human Services. Guidelines implementation panel report for: expert panel report 3-guidelines for the diagnosis and management of asthma. Partners putting guidelines into action. 2008; NIH Publication No. 09–6147.
22. Nkoy F, Fassl B, Wolfe D, et al. Sustaining compliance with pediatric asthma inpatient quality measures. AMIA Annu Symp Proc 2010;2010:547–51.
23. Kwok R, Dinh M, Dinh D, et al. Improving adherence to asthma clinical guidelines and discharge documentation from emergency departments: implementation of a dynamic and integrated electronic decision support system. Emerg Med Australas 2009;21(1):31–7.
24. Bell LM, Grundmeier R, Localio R, et al. Electronic health record-based decision support to improve asthma care: a cluster-randomized trial. Pediatrics 2010; 125(4):e770–7.
25. Boulet L, FitzGerald JM, Levy M, et al. A guide to the translation of the Global Initiative for Asthma (GINA) strategy into improved care. Eur Respir J 2012; 39(5):1220–9.
26. Alvanzo AH, Cohen GM, Nettleman M. Changing physician behavior: half-empty or half-full? Clin Govern Int J 2003;8(1):69–78.

Asthma Action Plans and Self-Management: Beyond the Traffic Light

Anna L. Edwards, NP-C, MSN

KEYWORDS

- Asthma action plan • Self-management • Health literacy • Outcomes • Measures
- Interventions

KEY POINTS

- Use of asthma action plans may be more effective in populations with a high use of services.
- Asthma outcome measures are variable but primarily focus on use.
- Asthma interventions should be appropriate for the population and/or the individual.

INTRODUCTION

Large health care organizations and health plans support care practices that incorporate self-management and action planning for the benefit of the patient and the potential savings in high-cost service use (emergency room/inpatient hospitalization). Smaller organizations and private practices are also incentivized as the health care industry emphasizes quality outcomes and financially compensates practitioners for meeting or exceeding quality benchmarks. Pay-for-performance is an example of a program that is "designed to offer financial incentives to physicians and other health care providers to meet defined quality, efficiency, or other targets," such as increasing the number of patients with asthma who are taking controller medications.[1]

Improving the care and management of chronic conditions, such as asthma, is a vital area of focus for individuals, providers, payers, and health systems. Because time and resources are limited in the care environment, it is important to identify what interventions are evidence-based, effective, and most plausible to implement. Clinicians and support staff must invest time in providing interventions that yield the best result and are appropriate for the population. Interventions that make practical sense may be difficult to implement in busy practice settings with multilevel challenges (ie, different individual patient educational needs).

Disclosure: The author has disclosed that she does not have any relationship with a commercial company that has a direct financial interest in the subject matter or materials discussed in the article or with a company making a competing product.
400 West Leadora Avenue, Glendora, CA 91741, USA
E-mail address: anedwards@dhs.lacounty.gov

ACTION PLANS

Action plans provide a guide for patients and families to self-manage chronic conditions, such as heart failure or asthma. Written action plans consist of 2 components: an algorithm consisting of clinical scenarios indicating the need to adjust medications or seek emergent medical care, and detailed information on the medication adjustment according to the clinical scenario.[2]

Asthma action plan templates are readily available through public and private professional medical organizations, and the use of these tools is supported by third-party payers. The National Asthma Education Prevention Program (NAEPP) Expert Panel Report 3 (EPR-3) recommends that every person diagnosed with asthma should have a written asthma action plan.[3] However, according to the National Health Interview Surveys (NHIS) information, one-third of all children and adults diagnosed with asthma here reported having a written asthma action plan.[4] Why is this the case? Some factors may include the length of time it takes to work on an action plan with a patient, or the complexity of the action plan tool may be a deterrent. The process of educating the patient may be time-consuming. With little or stretched staffing resources, extra time is a precious commodity. Perhaps providers lack the confidence that patients can follow an action plan.

Asthma action plans are used as a tool to support self-management of the condition. These plans provide concrete indicators for changes in health status with the steps/actions to make improvements. In asthma action plans, indicators of change in respiratory status are measured using peak flow meter performance figures (percentage ranges of personal best) or defined symptoms (eg, cough, shortness of breath).

However, asthma action plans are not necessarily the most appropriate tool for all patients with asthma. Lefevre and colleagues[2] suggest that perhaps the most appropriate population to develop an action plan is the high users of services. Although written asthma action plans may be appropriate for some patients, this intervention involves a significant time investment on the clinician's part and a level of confidence that patients understand how to use the plan. The use of a written asthma action plan alone does not demonstrate a significant improvement in several outcome measures, such as health care resource use, despite the wide support for use.[2]

Review of the current literature relating written asthma action plans to specific outcome measures provides relevant information on what intervention is most appropriate for patients. The literature examines the effect of asthma intervention variables on key outcome measures (**Box 1**).

Research and meta-analytic review identifies promising interventions or combinations of interventions that positively influence key asthma outcome measures. The remainder of this article highlights the following interventions derived from the literature: self-management education and asthma education that considers the patient's health literacy level.

SELF-MANAGEMENT EDUCATION

The area of self-management is a growing and widely recognized health promotion skill, particularly in chronic disease management. The skills needed for effective self-management must be cultivated and developed on both the provider and patient sides. The provider must learn to focus the care plan around what the patient views as their most important problem (collaboration), which is a shift from the ingrained medical model wherein the plan of care is designed around the medical facts and available treatments. The patient side of self-management is learning problem-solving skills that can

---

Box 1
Effect of asthma intervention variables on key outcome measures

Common asthma outcome measures in the literature

- Health care utilization (emergency room/hospitalization)
- Quality of life
- Medication adherence
- Frequency of rescue inhaler use
- Symptom control
- Missed work/school
- Functional status

Variables influencing the outcome measures

- Written action plan
- Peak flow meter use
- Asthma education
- Provider review
- Health literacy
- Self-management education

---

be applied to their personal health care issues.[5] Asthma-specific self-management education, such as trigger avoidance, medication use, and recognition of asthma control indicators, becomes more meaningful when patients are empowered with the skills to problem solve and have the support from their health care provider or team. A systematic review of research studies on educational and behavioral interventions for asthma suggests that a combined approach that includes self-management and regular communication between the patient and provider or clinical team have the "greatest effect on most outcomes."[6] The confidence that accompanies self-management education and skills can be the basis for complimentary interventions or tools, such as using written action plans or symptom recognition to make the decision to self-adjust medications.[7]

The Cochrane Collaboration's review of multiple study results on adult patients with asthma and the effects of self-management education and regular provider review versus usual care[8] on multiple outcome measures reinforces practitioner–patient skills and effort in asthma care interventions. Regularly scheduled practitioner follow-up for asthma care and monitoring of self-management behaviors yielded decreased use of acute services and improvement in asthma symptoms (nocturnal) and perceived quality of life.

HEALTH LITERACY–BASED ASTHMA EDUCATION

Patient-centered/focused care is a major health care focus in today's times. Developing a patient-centered clinical practice involves changes to access and new approaches to care delivery, such as taking into consideration the patient's health beliefs and understanding of health and illness.[9] Patient understanding, and therefore their ability to grasp information or important skills such as self-management education about their condition, depends on their health literacy. Health literacy is defined in

Healthy People 2010 as "The degree to which individuals have the capacity to obtain, process, and understand basic health information and services needed to make appropriate health decisions."[10] The level of health literacy is not, however, measured in the number of years of formal education or reading level.

Studies focused on asthma health literacy levels have shown relationships between low health literacy levels and increased asthma severity, functional level, perceived quality of life, and higher resource use.[11] Additionally, depressive symptoms may be higher in individuals with low health literacy according to Mancuso and Rincon's[11] review of related research studies.

For a patient to learn skills such as self-management, the level of health literacy should be evaluated and an individualized approach to improving the level should be designed. Where does a practitioner begin with this task? A resource such as the Office of Disease Prevention and Health Promotion offers information on health literacy basics and supporting research that is helpful for the interested practitioner. A starting point is to evaluate patients with chronic conditions, such as asthma, about their understanding of the condition and treatment. Tailoring an individualized education plan can pave the way for future self-management development skills, which has been shown to have a positive effect on multiple outcome measures.[12] Increasing practitioner awareness of support options, such as a health plan or community programs, is another important step in improving the supporting health literacy in the clinic practice.

DISCUSSION

A need exists for future studies to isolate the intervention variables and replicate the studies across populations to generalize the result findings. Self-management programs show a positive impact on chronic condition care, such as asthma. However, wide variations in program approaches make best practices difficult to isolate in the available literature. It would be valuable for future studies to test specific aspects of asthma self-management education relative to health literacy levels.

REFERENCES

1. Agency for Healthcare Research and Quality Web site. Available at: http://www.ahrq.gov/qual/pay4per.htm. Accessed July 30, 2012.
2. Lefevre F, Piper MP, Weiss K, et al. Do written action plans improve patient outcomes in asthma? An evidence-based analysis. J Fam Pract 2002;51(10):842–8.
3. National Institutes of Health, National Heart, Lung, Blood Institute (NHLBI). Guidelines for the diagnosis and management of asthma (EPR-3). Available at: http://www.nhlbi.nih.gov/guidelines/astha/asthgdln.pdf. Accessed August 8, 2012.
4. Centers for Disease Control and Prevention (CDC) website. Available at: http://www.cdc.gov/mmwr/preview/mmwrhtml/mm6017a4.htm?s_cid=mm6017a4_w. Accessed July 23, 2012.
5. Bodenheimer T, Lorig K, Holman H, et al. Patient self-management of chronic disease in primary care. JAMA 2002;288(19):2469–75.
6. Clark NM, Griffiths C, Keteyian SR, et al. Educational and behavioral interventions for asthma: who achieves which outcomes? A systematic review. J Asthma Allergy 2010;3:187–97.
7. Powell H, Gibson PG. Options for self-management education for adults with asthma. Cochrane Database Syst Rev 2002;(1):CD004107.

8. Gibson PG, Powell H, Wilson A, et al. Self-management education and regular practitioner review for adults with asthma. Cochrane Database Syst Rev 2003;(1):CD001117.
9. Bergeson SC, Dean JD. A systems approach to patient-centered care. JAMA 2006;296(23):2848–51.
10. National Network of Libraries of Medicine. Available at: http://nnlm.gov/outreach/consumer/hlthlit.html. Accessed July 23, 2012.
11. Mancuso CA, Rincon M. Impact of health literacy on longitudinal asthma outcomes. J Gen Intern Med 2006;21:813–7.
12. Janson SL, McGrath KW, Covington JK, et al. Individualized asthma self-management improves medication adherence and markers of asthma control. J Allergy Clin Immunol 2009;123(4):840–6.

A Systematic Review of Complementary and Alternative Medicine for Asthma Self-management

Maureen George, PhD, RN, AE-C[a,b],*, Maxim Topaz, RN, MA[c,d]

KEYWORDS

- Asthma • Self-management • Patient-provider communication
- Complementary and alternative medicine • Mind-body • Natural products • Disclosure

KEY POINTS

- There is wide patient support for the use of complementary and alternative medicine (CAM) as part of a comprehensive asthma self-management plan for both children and adults.
- The most popular complementary and alternative treatments for asthma fall broadly into the domains of natural products, mind-body medicine, and manipulative and body-based practices.
- Little empiric evidence to support the use of CAM can be gleaned from this systematic review because of both the small number of studies and the methodological weaknesses of the studies.
- Most complementary approaches reported by children and adults with asthma would be classified by the National Center for Complementary and Alternative Medicine as "likely safe" and "effectiveness unknown" or "likely ineffective."
- Rare but serious side effects have been reported with CAM for asthma self-management.
- Risky behaviors associated with CAM use for asthma include the substitution of complementary therapies for both "rescue" short-acting β-2 agonists and inhaled corticosteroids. These behaviors may add to unnecessary delays in seeking timely and appropriate medical intervention, thus contributing to excessive morbidity.
- There is suboptimal patient-provider communication about CAM use because of the failure of health care professionals to inquire about use and because of patients' reluctance to disclose use.
- To address patient preference for integrative care (concomitant use of CAM and prescription therapies) will require that clinicians conduct a more comprehensive assessment of use, be better informed about safety and risk of different therapies, and create a safe environment that fosters disclosure and shared decision making.

Funding Sources: Mr Topaz: None; Dr George: This study was supported by the National Center for Complementary and Alternative Medicine (National Institutes of Health) 1K23AT003907-01A1.
Conflict of Interest: None.
[a] Department of Family and Community Health, University of Pennsylvania School of Nursing, 418 Curie Boulevard, Philadelphia, PA 19104, USA; [b] Center for Clinical Epidemiology and Biostatistics (CCEB), Department of Biostatistics and Epidemiology, Perelman School of Medicine, 837 Blockley Hall, 423 Guardian Drive, Philadelphia, PA 19104-6021, USA; [c] University of Haifa, The Cheryl Spencer Department of Nursing Haifa, Mount Carmel 31905, Haifa, Israel; [d] University of Pennsylvania School of Nursing, 418 Curie Boulevard, Philadelphia, PA 19104, USA
* Corresponding author.
E-mail address: mgeorge@nursing.upenn.edu

Nurs Clin N Am 48 (2013) 53–149
http://dx.doi.org/10.1016/j.cnur.2012.11.002
0029-6465/13/$ – see front matter © 2013 Elsevier Inc. All rights reserved.

INTRODUCTION AND BACKGROUND

It has been more than 3 decades since Arthur Kleinman first reminded clinicians that individuals have more options to treat illness than just conventional biomedical approaches.[1] In fact, the health care professional is often the last resort for patients, consulted only after popular remedies and traditional healing methods have been exhausted.[2] To that end, it is estimated that as much as 80% of the world's health care is nonbiomedical.[3]

Although traditional healing is frequently integrated into the national medical system of its endemic country (eg, Ayurveda in India) and is common in places where limited access or prohibitive costs prevent the widespread adoption of biomedicine,[3] traditional healing is not an integral component of the North American health care systems. This has led to its characterization as "complementary" or "alternative" medicine. The term *complementary* describes traditional practices used in combination with conventional biomedical approaches, whereas *alternative* connotes traditional practices that replace or substitute for biomedicine.[4] The goal for many is *integrated* care in which the best treatments from conventional biomedical approaches are combined with safe and effective complementary and alternative medicine (CAM).[4]

The National Center for Complementary and Alternative Medicine (NCCAM), the leading federal CAM research agency in the United States, defines CAM as a variety of medical systems, healing traditions, and products not typically considered to be part of conventional biomedical approaches.[4] As seen in **Table 1**, CAM can be broadly characterized into domains that include whole medical systems, natural products, manipulative and body-based practices, movement therapies, traditional healers, and energy field healing. Although useful for purposes of grouping, the clinician must remember that a CAM approach may overlap with several domains.

Despite growing interest in integrated care,[5] much of CAM continues to be delivered outside of the North American health care systems at a considerable out-of-pocket cost.[6] In fact, US adults are more likely to use CAM when conventional medical care is unaffordable.[7] Despite these costs, CAM is widely used. Nationwide surveys suggest that three-quarters of US[7] and Canadian adults[5,8] have used some form of CAM in their lifetime. In addition, although there are no national data on CAM use in Mexico, a systematic review indicates high rates of indigenous Mexican CAM use among Mexican-American adults.[9]

Frequently, CAM use is reported to be highest among well-educated higher-income white adults.[7] However, this is likely a function of survey questions that focus on vitamins and herb ingestion, and body-based (massage, chiropractic care) and mind-body therapies (yoga, acupuncture) to the exclusion of folk medicine and prayer, which are CAMs more commonly used by people of color and by the poor. For example, when folk medicine (defined as a "range of remedies including prayer, healing touch or laying on of hands, charms, herbal teas or tinctures, magic rituals") was included in the 2002 National Health Interview Survey (NHIS), CAM prevalence was highest in black and Hispanic individuals and those living in poverty.[10] Nonvitamin, nonmineral natural products and deep-breathing exercises were the most commonly reported CAM[7] after prayer[10] among US adults, whereas chiropractic care, massage, relaxation techniques, and prayer were most common among Canadian adults.[5] In both groups, CAM was used for the treatment of a variety of somatic and psychiatric complaints, including neck, back, and joint discomfort; upper respiratory infections; anxiety; and depression.[5,7]

CAM is also frequently used by or for children. The 2006 Fraser Institute[5] and 2007 NHIS[7] surveys were the first comprehensive national surveys directed at

Table 1
CAM domains and examples

NCCAM Domain Definitions	CAM Type	Examples	NCCAM Definition/Description
Whole Medical Systems are complete systems of theory and practice that have evolved over time in different cultures and apart from Western medicine	Ayurveda		Developed in India, it aims to integrate the body, mind, and spirit to prevent and treat disease using herbs, diet, massage, and yoga.
	Naturopathy		Developed in Europe, naturopathy seeks to stimulate self-healing through the use of dietary and lifestyle changes used in concert with massage, herbs and joint manipulation.
	Traditional Chinese Medicine (TCM)		Developed in China, TCM is based on the belief that disease is the result of an imbalance in yin and yang and disrupted flow of qi (life force). Balance and flow can be restored through the use of herbs, acupuncture, meditation, and massage.
	Homeopathy		Developed in Europe, homeopathy seeks to stimulate self-healing through doses of highly diluted substances that in larger doses would produce the symptoms of concern ("like cures like").
Natural Products are substances produced by living organisms and built by cells from sugars, amino acids, and so forth	Botanicals	Herbs and herbal products	Products that include any plant-based component.
	Minerals	Calcium, folate, iron, magnesium, selenium, zinc	
	Specialized diets	Gluten-free, allergen-free, ketogenic, low-residue	A special diet in which foods that produce unwanted symptoms are avoided.
	Dietary supplements	Minerals, vitamins, herbs, enzymes, proteins, organ tissues, or glands and metabolites	Any product taken by mouth with the intent of supplementing the diet.
	Vitamins	A, B12, B6, C, D, E, K	
	Herbs and herbal preparations	Echinacea, St Johns wort, chamomile, ginseng	Plants with leaves, seeds, flowers, bark, or roots used for medicinal purposes.
	Probiotics	Live microorganisms (bacteria; yeast)	

(continued on next page)

Table 1
(continued)

NCCAM Domain Definitions	CAM Type	Examples	NCCAM Definition/Description
Mind-body Medicine	Meditation	Transcendental, Mindfulness	Meditation teaches an individual to focus attention, to become mindful of thoughts, feelings, and sensations and to observe them in a nonjudgmental way. Meditation is performed to achieve calmness, relaxation, and psychological balance.
	Tai chi		Developed in China as a martial art, tai chi is a "moving meditation" in which practitioners move their bodies slowly, gently, and with awareness, while breathing deeply.
	Guided imagery	Mental imagery, visualization	In guided imagery, the individual focuses on pleasant images or is led through storytelling or visualizations to replace negative or stressful feelings for the purpose of promoting relaxation.
	Relaxation	Progressive muscle relaxation, passive muscle relaxation, relaxation breathing	In this practice, the individual focuses on tightening and relaxing each muscle group. It is often combined with guided imagery and breathing exercises.
	Hypnosis		Phrases or nonverbal cues (called a "suggestion") produce relaxation to relieve pain and anxiety.
	Qi gong		Similar to tai chi.
	Yoga	Hatha, Iyengar, Ashtanga, Vinyasa, Bikram	Originating in ancient Indian philosophy, yoga combines physical postures, breathing techniques, and meditation or relaxation.
	Art therapy		Art-making as a therapeutic process.
	Cognitive behavioral therapy		Psychotherapeutic method to reduce stress and anxiety.
	Acupuncture		Part of traditional Chinese medicine (TCM), acupuncture aims to restore and maintain health through the stimulation of specific points on the body to encourage the flow of qi through channels called meridians.
	Biofeedback		Electronic devices are used to teach individuals to consciously reduce stress.
	Breathing retraining	Buteyko breathing exercises	Nasal breathing, reduced breathing, and relaxation are used to "normalize" breathing.
	Journaling		Writing therapy.

Category	Technique	Description
	Music therapy	Use of music to promote well-being or promote relaxation.
	Humoral balance	Ancient theory that disease results from an imbalance of 4 "humors." Application of hot-cold therapies can be traced to this belief system.
	Deep breathing	Conscious slowing of breathing by focusing on taking regular and deep breaths to promote relaxation.
Manipulative and Body-based Practices focus primarily on the structures and systems of the body	Spinal manipulation — Chiropractic care, Craniosacral therapy (cranial osteopathy)	The application of a controlled force to the joint by use of hands or a device with the intent of reducing pain and/or improving physical functioning.
	Massage — Swedish, shiatsu, Acupressure, Trager, Craniosacral therapy (cranial osteopathy)	Blood flow and oxygen are increased to the massaged area by pressing, rubbing, and moving soft tissues with the hands and fingers. The intent of massage is to reduce pain and stress and enhance relaxation, mood, and general well-being.
Movement Therapies include Eastern and Western movement-based practices to promote physical, mental, emotional, and spiritual well-being	Pilates	A physical fitness approach to core training that uses apparatuses to apply resistance as well as props, such as weighted balls.
	Rolfing	Deep fascial tissue manipulation and movement used to reduce stress by bringing the body into proper alignment with gravity.
	Alexander technique (AT)	This technique aims to teach individuals to stand and move free of tension. AT is not an exercise or relaxation program.
Traditional Healers use indigenous and religious knowledge, beliefs, and experiences to treat disease and promote health	Shaman, Curandero, Santero, Houngan, Mambos	Healing power is passed down through generations via oral transmission and apprenticeships. Its use is generally reserved for members of a regional or cultural community.
Energy Field Healing involves the manipulation of the subtle energy fields imbued in humans	Magnet therapy	Magnets produce magnetic fields that are proposed to reduce pain.
	Reiki — Energy-field manipulation	Healing of the body and the spirit can be facilitated by the practitioner's transmitting universal energy to the person from a distance or from placing their hands on or near the individual.
	Light therapy	Exposure to green and blue wavelength light to promote sleep.
	Therapeutic touch	Manipulation of energy fields by placing hands on, or near, an individual.

Abbreviations: CAM, complementary and alternative medicine; NCCAM, National Center for Complementary and Alternative Medicine.

understanding CAM use among North American children. Caregivers of children aged 0 to 17 were interviewed about the child's CAM use. Twelve percent of US[7] and 15% of Canadian youth[5] reported CAM use in the prior 12 months to treat neck and back pain, anxiety, and attention deficit and hyperactivity disorders, as well as head and chest colds.[7] Children were most likely to use nonvitamin, nonmineral natural products, chiropractic care,[5,7] homeopathy, and acupuncture.[11] CAM use was fivefold higher in children who had a CAM-using parent compared with children who did not.[7]

Complementary and Alternative Medicine for Asthma

Although CAM is commonly used to maintain wellness, national surveys have demonstrated their extensive use in treating common chronic medical conditions, including lung and digestive disorders, heart disease, hypertension, and diabetes.[5,7] Lung problems generally[5] and asthma and allergies specifically[5,7,10] rank in the top 15 most common medical conditions for which CAM is used for both children and adults. Unfortunately, there is a lack of recent literature summarizing the rates of CAM use among children and adults with asthma. Moreover, there is a critical need to compile and summarize the growing body of evidence on the most prevalent CAM modalities used, CAM effectiveness, and its possible side effects. This summary is crucial for allopathic and CAM practitioners treating patients with asthma, as well as individuals with asthma and their families who are engaged in decision making regarding asthma self-management practices.

The aim of this systematic review was twofold. First, we aimed to quantitatively summarize the existing body of research on CAM use for asthma among children and adults. Second, we wanted to reflect on the most frequent CAM modalities used, the methodological quality and patterns presented in CAM studies, and the potential benefits and dangers of CAM use in asthma.

METHODS

A systematic review of the literature[12] was conducted using the following databases: PubMed, PyscINFO, and SCOPUS. The following search terms were used: "asthma" AND "complementary medicine," "alternative medicine," "complementary and alternative medicine," "herbs," "diet," "dietary supplements," "vitamins," "acupuncture," "breathing (Buteyko) exercises," "relaxation," "mind-body," "homeopathy," "ayurveda," "traditional Chinese medicine," "colon cleansing," "music," "chiropractic," "massage," "art therapy," "aromatherapy," "yoga," "tai-chi." Search terms were determined after reviewing existing CAM literature, reviewing information from NCCAM and compiling associated keywords and subject headings. **Table 1** summarizes the different CAM domains and examples.

The place of publication was limited to North America (Canada, Mexico, and the United States). Publications were also limited to English, Spanish, and French languages. We did not limit the age of publications. Manuscripts were included if they (1) presented primary or original research and (2) were focused on CAM use among children and adults with asthma. Manuscripts were excluded if they were duplicates from different databases or did not present original research on CAM use among individuals with asthma.

Data Collection and Analyses

The two authors (M.T. and M.G.) independently reviewed the abstracts and articles for inclusion with 100% interrater reliability. Data were extracted using a standardized template developed by the researchers to capture all relevant data. The template was reviewed by the authors and consensus reached through discussion between the authors.

STUDY FINDINGS
Search Results

A total of 1960 abstracts were identified from the initial review, of which 904 were duplicates. After a detailed review, 984 additional articles were excluded because they did not meet the inclusion criteria: 322 articles did not directly focus on CAM use among individuals with asthma; 214 manuscripts did not present original research; and 448 of the studies were conducted outside of the United States, Canada, or Mexico. As a result, 72 articles were included in the review. See **Fig. 1** for the detailed description of the search process and findings and **Table 2** presenting qualitative summary of the reviewed articles.

In general, there is an increasing body of research on the use of different CAM modalities among individuals with asthma. As presented in **Fig. 2**, the number of articles on the topic remained low until the mid 1990s and then grew steadily, especially through the past decade.

Methodological Issues

Overall, the reviewed literature includes studies conducted using diverse designs and methodological techniques, ranging from randomized controlled trials (RCTs) to

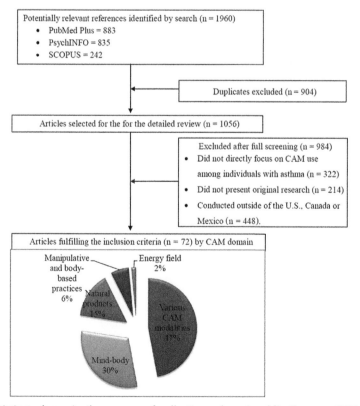

Fig. 1. Distinct phases in the process of collecting relevant publications on CAM use for asthma and their results.

Table 2
Summary of included articles: CAM use in asthma

Authors, Primary	Design	Population	Results	Conclusions	Categories/Domain
Knoeller et al,[15] 2012	Survey, correlational	27,927 employed adults with current work-related asthma (WRA) as presented in the 2006–2008 Behavioral Risk Factor Surveillance System Asthma Call-Back Survey from 37 states and the District of Columbia.	An estimated 56.6% of individuals with WRA reported using CAM compared with 27.9% of those with non-WRA (PR = 2.0). People with WRA were more likely than those with non-WRA to have adverse asthma events including an asthma attack in the past month (PR = 1.43), urgent treatment for worsening asthma (PR = 1.74), emergency room visit (PR = 1.95), overnight hospital stay (PR = 2.49), and poorly controlled asthma (PR = 1.27). The associations of WRA with adverse asthma events remained after stratifying for CAM use.	Individuals with WRA were more likely to use CAM to control their asthma. However, there was no evidence that the use of CAM modified the association of WRA with adverse asthma events.	Adults; various CAM modalities

| Luberto et al,[60] 2012 | Survey, correlational | 282 adolescents (Time 1: n = 151, Time 2: n = 131) completed self-report measures | Participants (M(age) = 15.8, SD = 1.85) were primarily African American (n = 129 [85%]) and female (n = 91 [60%]) adolescents with asthma. High and low CAM users differed significantly in terms of several psychosocial health outcomes, both cross-sectionally and longitudinally. In cross-sectional multivariable analyses, greater frequency of praying was associated with better psychosocial health-related quality of life. No longitudinal relationships remained significant in multivariable analyses. | Specific CAM techniques are differentially associated with psychosocial outcomes, indicating the importance of examining CAM modalities individually. When controlling for key covariates, CAM use was not associated with psychosocial outcomes over time. Further research should examine the effects of CAM use in controlled research settings. | Adolescents; various CAM modalities |

(continued on next page)

Table 2
(continued)

Authors, Primary	Design	Population	Results	Conclusions	Categories/Domain
Philp et al,[105] 2012	Survey, correlational (retrospective cohort study)	187 children prescribed daily medications for all 3 y of the study	Patients had high rates of adherence. The mean percent missed asthma daily controller medication doses per week was 7.7% (SD = 14.2%). Medication Adherence Scale scores (range: 4–20, with lower scores reflecting higher adherence) had an overall mean of 7.5 (SD = 2.9). In multivariate analyses, controlling for demographic factors and asthma severity, initiation of CAM use was not associated with subsequent adherence (P>.05).	The data from this study suggest that CAM use is not necessarily "competitive" with conventional asthma therapies; families may incorporate different health belief systems simultaneously in their asthma management. As CAM use becomes more prevalent, it is important for physicians to ask about CAM use in a nonjudgmental fashion.	Adolescent; Children; various CAM modalities

| Shen and Oraka,[16] 2012 | Survey, correlational | 5435 children from the Asthma Call Back Survey (ACBS) 2006–2008, were included in this analysis. | Overall, 26.7% of children with current asthma reported CAM use in the previous 12 mo. Among them, the 3 most commonly used therapies were breathing techniques, vitamins, and herbal products. Multivariate analysis of CAM use revealed higher adjusted odds ratios (aOR) among children who experienced cost barriers to conventional health care compared with children with no cost barrier (aOR = 1.8). Children with poorly controlled asthma were most likely to use all types of CAM when compared with their counterparts with well-controlled asthma: aOR = 2.3 for any CAM; aOR = 1.7 for self-care based CAM; and aOR = 4.4 for practitioner-based CAM. | Children with poorly controlled asthma are more likely to use CAM; this likelihood persists after controlling for other factors (including parent's education, barriers to conventional health care, and controller medication use). CAM is also more commonly used by children who experienced cost barriers to conventional asthma care. CAM use could be a marker to identify patients who need patient/family education and support and thus facilitate improved asthma control. | Children; various CAM modalities |

(continued on next page)

Table 2
(continued)

Authors, Primary	Design	Population	Results	Conclusions	Categories/Domain
Cotton et al,[33] 2011	Survey, correlational	151 adolescents with asthma recruited from a children's hospital completed questionnaires addressing demographic and clinical variables and 10 CAM modalities.	Participants' mean age was 15.8 (SD = 1.8), 60% were female, and 85% were African American. Seventy-one percent reported using CAM for symptom management in the past month. Relaxation (64%) and prayer (61%) were the most frequently reported modalities and were perceived to be the most efficacious. Adolescents most commonly reported considering using relaxation (85%) and prayer (80%) for future symptom management. Participants were most likely to disclose their use of yoga (59%) and diet (57%), and least likely to disclose prayer (33%) and guided	Many urban adolescents used and would consider using CAM, specifically relaxation and prayer, for asthma symptom management. African Americans, older adolescents, and those with more frequent symptoms were more likely to use and/or consider using CAM. Providers caring for urban adolescents with asthma should discuss CAM with patients, particularly those identified as likely to use CAM. Future studies should examine relationships between CAM use and health outcomes.	Adolescents; various CAM modalities

			imagery (36%) to providers. In multivariable analyses, older adolescents (OR = 1.27, $P<.05$) and African Americans (OR = 2.76, $P<.05$) were more likely to use relaxation. Adolescents with more frequent asthma symptoms (OR = 0.98, $P<.05$) were more likely to use prayer. African Americans were more likely to report using prayer (OR = 3.47, $P<.05$) and consider using prayer (OR = 7.98, $P<.01$) in the future for symptom management.		
Kligler et al,[23] 2011	Prospective parallel group repeated measurement randomized study	154 patients were randomized and included in the intention-to-treat analysis (77 control, 77 treatment).	Treatment participants showed greater improvement than controls at 6 mo for the Asthma Quality of Life Questionnaire total score ($P<.001$) and for 3 subscales, Activity ($P<.001$), Symptoms ($P = .02$), and Emotion ($P<.001$).	A low-cost group-oriented integrative medicine intervention can lead to significant improvement in quality of life in adults with asthma.	Adults; yoga (mind-body); dietary supplements (natural products); journaling (mind-body)

(continued on next page)

Table 2
(continued)

Authors, Primary	Design	Population	Results	Conclusions	Categories/Domain
Long et al,[63] 2011	Intervention trial (feasibility study with 2 intervention groups)	Cohort 1 (n = 11) was recruited from the community and attended intervention sessions at an urban university. Cohort 2 (n = 7) was school based and recruited from an African American charter school.	The intervention was rated as highly acceptable by participating families. Feasibility was much stronger for the school-based than the university-based recruitment mechanism. Initial efficacy data suggest that both cohorts showed preintervention to postintervention improvements in lung function, perceived stress, and depressed mood.	Findings provide evidence for the feasibility of offering asthma-related stress-management training in a school setting. Initial findings offer support for future, large-scale efficacy studies.	Children; relaxation and biofeedback (mind-body)

Mithani and Monteleone,[109] 2011	Survey, descriptive (pilot)	181 individuals with asthma filled out the survey	Over a period of 14 mo, 18% of the patients completing a survey reported using alternative therapies to treat asthma. The most common alternative therapy used was exercise/massage; the least popular was homeopathy. The highest users were women (59%), ages 41–50 (31%), white ethnicity (63%), higher education (56%), and higher annual household income (84%). The major reasons for usage were having more control of their health, personal beliefs, and concern over side effects of conventional medication.	The rate of alternative therapy use in patients with asthma in central New Jersey was lower than in some other studies. It is important for physicians to take CAM therapies into account to develop a health care plan consistent with patients' beliefs and expectations.	Adults; various CAM modalities

(continued on next page)

Table 2
(continued)

Authors, Primary	Design	Population	Results	Conclusions	Categories/Domain
Wechsler et al,[80] 2011	Randomized controlled trial (pilot)	46 patients with asthma were randomized to active treatment with an albuterol inhaler, a placebo inhaler, sham acupuncture, or no intervention.	Albuterol resulted in a 20% increase in FEV(1), as compared with approximately 7% with each of the other 3 interventions ($P<.001$). However, patients' reports of improvement after the intervention did not differ significantly for the albuterol inhaler (50% improvement), placebo inhaler (45%), or sham acupuncture (46%), but the subjective improvement with all 3 of these interventions was significantly greater than that with the no-intervention control (21%) ($P<.001$).	Although albuterol, but not the 2 placebo interventions, improved FEV(1) in these patients with asthma, albuterol provided no incremental benefit with respect to the self-reported outcomes. Placebo effects can be clinically meaningful and can rival the effects of active medication in patients with asthma. However, from a clinical-management and research-design perspective, patient self-reports can be unreliable. An assessment of untreated responses in asthma may be essential in evaluating patient-reported outcomes.	Adults; acupuncture (mind-body)

| Zayas et al,[47] 2011 | Qualitative, semistructured individual interviews | 30 Puerto Rican adults who had asthma or were caregivers of children with asthma were interviewed in person. | Participants identified 75 ethnomedical treatments for asthma. Behavioral strategies that included conventional care (environmental remediation) and folk beliefs (chihuahuas in the home cure/control asthma) were significantly more likely to be used or perceived effective compared with ingested and topical remedies ($P<.001$). Among information sources for ingested and topical remedies, those recommended by community members were significantly less likely to be used or perceived to be effective ($P<.001$) compared with other sources. | Study sample of Puerto Rican subjects with a regular source of medical care was significantly more likely to use or perceive as effective behavioral strategies compared with ingested and topical remedies. Allopathic clinicians should ask Puerto Rican patients about their use of ethnomedical therapies for asthma to better understand their health beliefs and to integrate ethnomedical therapies with allopathic medicine. | Adults and caregivers of children with asthma; ethnomedical therapies; various CAM modalities |

(continued on next page)

Table 2
(continued)

Authors, Primary	Design	Population	Results	Conclusions	Categories/Domain
Beebe et al,[71] 2010	Randomized controlled trial	22 children with asthma were randomized to an active art therapy or wait-list control group.	Score changes from baseline to completion of art therapy indicated (1) improved problem-solving and affect drawing scores; (2) improved worry, communication, and total quality of life scores; and (3) improved Beck anxiety and self-concept scores in the active group relative to the control group. At 6 mo, the active group maintained some positive changes relative to the control group, including (1) drawing affect scores, (2) the worry and quality of life scores, and (3) the Beck anxiety score. Frequency of asthma exacerbations before and after the 6-mo study interval did not differ between the 2 groups.	This was the first randomized trial demonstrating that children with asthma receive benefit from art therapy that includes decreased anxiety and increased quality of life.	Children; art therapy

| Covar et al,[24] 2010 | Randomized controlled trial | 43 children with mild to moderate persistent asthma were randomized to receive daily novel nutritional formula (n = 23) or control formula (n = 20) for 12 wk. | Daily consumption of either NNF (a nutritional supplement composed of antioxidants, omega-3 and omega-6 fatty acids) or a control formula showed improvement in asthma-free days over time but there was no difference between groups. However, the NNF group had lower exhaled nitric oxide levels compared with the control group at weeks 4, 8, and 12 (P<.05). An overall group difference in log FEV(1) PC 20 (P = .05) was found in favor of the NNF group as well. Significantly higher levels of EPA in plasma (P<.01) and peripheral blood mononuclear cell (PBMC) (P<.01) phospholipids in the NNF group compared with the control group within 2 wk indicated good adherence with daily NNF intake. There were no differences in adverse events for NNF vs control groups after 12 wk. | Both NNF and control groups demonstrated improvement in asthma-free days. The NNF-treated group had reduced biomarkers of disease activity. Rapid PBMC fatty acid composition changes reflected an anti-inflammatory profile. Dietary supplementation with NNF was safe and well tolerated. | Children; dietary supplements (natural products) |

(continued on next page)

Table 2
(continued)

Authors, Primary	Design	Population	Results	Conclusions	Categories/Domain
Joubert et al,[13] 2010	Survey, correlational study	3327 responses of those ever having asthma as presented in National Health Interview Survey (NHIS) were analyzed	Overall CAM use differed significantly by asthma status, with 49% of those with asthma episodes using CAM compared with 42% of those who did not have an episode in the past year. Self-care–based therapies were more likely to be used than practitioner-based therapies by individuals with a single comorbid condition compared with those with 2 or more comorbidities.	Although this study supports previous work indicating that disease severity (in this instance, asthma within the past year) is significantly associated with CAM use, it did not support studies showing greater CAM use in the presence of a greater number of comorbidities, suggesting that disease burden is a limiting factor when it comes to self-care–based CAM use.	Adults; various CAM modalities
Kapoor et al,[65] 2010	Intervention-follow-up trial	3 participants	At the onset of the intervention, it was found that lung functioning, particularly FEV(1) increased in all 3 participants, with effect sizes ranging from –0.32 to –2.48. FEF25-75 improved in one of the participants. In addition, a positive	School-based relaxation and guided imagery intervention improved anxiety and lung functioning.	Children; relaxation and guided imagery (mind-body)

				impact was also seen in the lowering of anxiety scores across all 3 participants, with effect sizes ranging from 0.12 to 1.69.	
Kazaks et al,[50] 2010	Randomized controlled trial	55 males and females aged 21–55 y with mild to moderate asthma according to the 2002 National Heart, Lung, and Blood Institute (NHLBI) and Asthma Education and Prevention Program (NAEPP) guidelines and who used only beta-agonists or inhaled corticosteroids (ICS) as asthma medications.	The concentration of methacholine required to cause a 20% drop in FEV(1) increased significantly from baseline to month 6 within the Mg group. Peak expiratory flow rate (PEFR) showed a 5.8% predicted improvement over time ($P = .03$) in those consuming the Mg. There was significant improvement in AQLQ mean score units ($P<.01$) and in overall ACQ score only in the Mg group ($P = .05$) after 6.5 mo of supplementation. Despite these improvements, there were no significant changes in any of the markers of Mg status.	Adults who received oral Mg supplements showed improvement in objective measures of bronchial reactivity to methacholine and PEFR and in subjective measures of asthma control and quality of life.	Adults; Mg diet supplements (natural products)

(continued on next page)

Table 2
(continued)

Authors, Primary	Design	Population	Results	Conclusions	Categories/Domain
MacRedmond et al,[51] 2010	Randomized controlled study	28 adult subjects with mild asthma were randomized to conjugated linoleic acid (CLA) 4.5 g/d or placebo for 12 wk in addition to usual treatment.	Subjects in the CLA (omega-6 fatty acid) group had a significant improvement in airway hyperresponsiveness at week 12 compared with week 0 (PC 20 6.6 [2.1] mg/mL vs 2.2 [0.7] mg/mL; $P<.05$). The CLA group had a significant reduction in weight and BMI compared with placebo and this was associated with a reduction in leptin/adiponectin ratio. There were no differences in systemic cytokine levels, induced sputum cell counts, quality-of-life scores, or adverse events.	Omega-6 fatty acid treatment as an adjunct to usual care in overweight mildly and moderately severe adults with asthma was well tolerated and was associated with improvements in airway hyperresponsiveness and BMI.	Adults; conjugated linoleic acid (natural products)

| Marino and Shen,[17] 2010 | Survey, correlational | 7352 responses from the 2006 Behavioral Risk Factor Surveillance System (BRFSS) data from a subset of 25 states that completed the follow-up Asthma Callback Survey. | The prevalence of CAM use among adults with asthma was 39.6% (95% confidence interval [CI] = 36.9–42.3). There was no significant association with CAM use by sex, race/ethnicity, age, education, or geographic region. After adjusting for demographics and region, CAM use was significantly higher among persons with (1) financial barriers to asthma care (odds ratio [OR] = 2.8, 95% CI = 1.9–4.1); (2) an emergency room (ER) visit due to asthma (OR = 1.7 95% CI = 1.1–2.6); and (3) ≥ 14 asthma-associated disability days during the previous year (OR = 2.1, 95% CI = 1.4–3.1). | CAM use is common among adults with asthma. It is associated with financial barriers to asthma care and poor asthma control. Physicians should discuss CAM use with their asthma patients. | Adults; various CAM modalities |

(continued on next page)

Table 2
(continued)

Authors, Primary	Design	Population	Results	Conclusions	Categories/Domain
Metcalfe et al,[8] 2010	Survey, correlational study	400,055 Canadians aged ≥12 between 2001–2005 as presented in the Canadian Community Health Survey	Weighted estimates show that 12.4% (95% CI: 12.2–12.5) of Canadians visited a CAM practitioner in the year they were surveyed; this rate was significantly higher for those with asthma 15.1% (95% CI: 14.5–15.7) and migraine 19.0% (95% CI: 18.4–19.6), and	A large proportion of Canadians use CAM services. Physicians should be aware that their patients may be accessing other services and should be prepared to ask and answer questions about the risks and benefits of CAM services in conjunction with standard medical care.	Adults; various CAM modalities

significantly lower for those with diabetes 8.0% (95% CI: 7.4–8.6), whereas the rate in those with epilepsy (10.3%, 95% CI: 8.4–12.2) was not significantly different from the general population.

(continued on next page)

Table 2
(continued)

Authors, Primary	Design	Population	Results	Conclusions	Categories/Domain
Sidora-Arcoleo et al,[119] 2010	Tool validation study	337 parents of children with asthma from Bronx and Rochester, NY.	Bronx parents were more likely to perceive their child's asthma to be moderate or severe than the Rochester parents. Bronx children were older and had longer duration of asthma and reported more acute health care visits (past year). Bronx parents reported total Asthma Illness Representation Scale scores more closely aligned with the lay model than Rochester parents. The Asthma Illness Representation Scale instrument demonstrated acceptable internal reliability among the Bronx sample (total score alpha = 0.82) and the Asthma Illness Representation Scale (AIRS) subscale Cronbach alpha coefficients were remarkably similar to	The AIRS instrument exhibited good internal reliability, external validity, and differentiated parents based on ethnicity, poverty, and education. Assessment of asthma IRs during the health care visit will allow the HCP and parent to discuss and negotiate a shared asthma management plan for the child, which will hopefully lead to improved medication adherence and asthma health outcomes.	Children; various CAM modalities

those obtained from the original validation study (range = 0.54–0.83). Poor parents and those with less than a high school education had lower total AIRS scores than their counterparts. White parents had AIRS scores more closely aligned with the professional model compared with each of the ethnic subgroups. A perception of less severe asthma, fewer reports of asthma and somatization symptoms, and a positive HCP relationship were associated with IRs congruent with the professional model. IRs aligned with the professional model were associated with fewer acute asthma-related health care visits.

(continued on next page)

Table 2
(continued)

Authors, Primary	Design	Population	Results	Conclusions	Categories/Domain
Torres-Llenza et al,[11] 2010	Survey, correlational	2027 children with asthma.	The median age of the 2027 children surveyed was 6.1 y (interquartile range 3.3–10.5 y); 58% were male and 59% of children had persistent asthma. The prevalence of CAM use was 13% (95% CI 12%–15%). Supplemental vitamins (24%), homeopathy (18%), and acupuncture (11%) were the most commonly reported CAMs. Multivariable logistic regression analysis confirmed the association of CAM use with age younger than 6 y (OR 1.86; 95% CI 1.20–2.96), Asian ethnicity (OR 1.89; 95% CI 1.01–3.52), episodic asthma (OR 1.88; 95% CI 1.08–3.28), and poor asthma control (OR 1.98; 95% CI 1.80–3.31).	The prevalence of reported CAM use among Quebec children with asthma remained modest (13%), with vitamins, homeopathy and acupuncture being the most popular modalities. CAM use was associated with preschool age, Asian ethnicity, episodic asthma, and poor asthma control.	Children; various CAM modalities

| Roy et al,[59] 2010 | Survey, correlational | 326 adults with persistent asthma who received care at 2 inner-city outpatient clinics. | Overall, 25.4% of patients reported herbal remedy use. Univariate analyses showed that herbal remedy use was associated with decreased ICS adherence and increased asthma morbidity. In multivariable analysis, herbal remedy use was associated with lower ICS adherence (OR, 0.4; 95%) after adjusting for confounders. Herbal remedy users were also more likely to worry about the adverse effects of ICS ($P = .01$). | The use of herbal remedies was associated with lower adherence to ICS and worse outcomes among inner-city asthmatic patients. Medication beliefs, such as worry about ICS adverse effects, may in part mediate this relationship. Physicians should routinely ask patients with asthma about CAM use, especially those whose asthma is poorly controlled. | Adults; herbs (natural products) |

(continued on next page)

Table 2
(continued)

Authors, Primary	Design	Population	Results	Conclusions	Categories/Domain
Birdee et al,[18] 2009	Survey, correlational	31,044 responses from the 2002 National Health Interview Survey (NHIS) Alternative Medicine Supplement.	We found that neither age nor sex was associated with T'ai chi and qigong use. T'ai chi and qigong users were more likely than nonusers to be Asian than white (OR 2.02, 95% CI 1.30–3.15), college educated (OR 2.44, 95% CI 1.97–3.03), and less likely to live in the Midwest (OR 0.64, 95% CI 0.42–0.96) or the southern United	In the United States, T'ai chi and qigong is practiced for health by a diverse population, and users report benefits for maintaining health.	Adults; T'ai chi (mind body); qigong (energy field)

States (OR 0.51, 95% CI 0.36–0.72) than the West. T'ai chi and qigong use was associated independently with higher reports of musculoskeletal conditions (OR 1.43, 95% CI 1.11–1.83), severe sprains (OR 1.65, 95% CI 1.14–2.40), and asthma (OR 1.50, 95% CI 1.08–2.10).

(continued on next page)

Table 2
(continued)

Authors, Primary	Design	Population	Results	Conclusions	Categories/Domain
George et al,[37] 2009	Qualitative, semi-structured individual interviews	25 adults (92% female; 76% African American; mean age 39)	Only 1 subject had received asthma self-management training and only 10 (40%) used short-acting beta-(2) agonist-based (SABA) self-management protocols for the early treatment of acute asthma. No subject used a peak flow meter or an asthma action plan. Most (52%) chose to initially treat acute asthma with CAM despite the availability of SABAs. Importantly, 21 (84%) preferred an integrated approach using both conventional and CAM treatments. Four themes associated with acute asthma	All patents' acute asthma self-management strategies should be evaluated for their timeliness and appropriateness. This would be of particular importance for vulnerable populations who bear a disproportionate burden of the disease and who have the fewest resources.	Adults; various CAM modalities

self-management emerged from the qualitative analysis. The first theme, safety, reflected subjects' perception that CAM was safer than SABA. Severity addressed the calculation that subjects made in determining if SABA or CAM was indicated based on the degree of symptoms they were experiencing. The third theme, speed and strength of the combination, described subjects' belief in the superiority of integrating CAM and SABA for acute asthma self-management. The final theme, sense of identity, spoke to the ability of CAM to provide a customized self-management strategy that subjects desired.

(continued on next page)

Table 2
(continued)

Authors, Primary	Design	Population	Results	Conclusions	Categories/Domain
Post-White et al,[35] 2009	Survey, descriptive	281 respondents participated in the survey	CAM use was higher in children with epilepsy (61.9%), cancer (59%), asthma (50.7%), and sickle cell disease (47.4%) than in general pediatrics (36%). Children most often used prayer (60.5%), massage (27.9%), specialty vitamins (27.2%), chiropractic care (25.9%), and dietary supplements (21.8%). Parents who used CAM for themselves (68.7%) were more likely to access CAM for their child. Most parents (62.6%) disclosed some or all of their child's use of CAM to providers.	Within the same geographic region, children with chronic and life-threatening illness use more CAM therapies than children seen in primary care clinics.	Children; various CAM modalities
Cabana et al,[32] 2008	Survey, correlational	1322 parents of children with asthma	Eleven percent (141/1322) of children used CAM. Parents of children on daily medications who were perceived to have poor asthma control were almost 3 times more likely to use CAM than parents of	Parent perception of asthma control is significantly associated with CAM use. It is important for providers to elicit information regarding CAM use in the clinic, as this may imply that the asthma	Children; various CAM modalities

			children on no daily medications who were perceived to have high asthma control (risk ratio: = 2.81; CI: 1.72–4.60); age, gender, race, income, and education level were not significant independent predictors.	symptoms may not be well controlled.	
Cowie et al,[79] 2008	Randomized controlled trial	129 individuals with asthma were randomized to 2 groups	Both groups showed substantial and similar improvement and a high proportion with asthma control 6 mo after completion of the intervention. In the Buteyko group the proportion with asthma control increased from 40% to 79% and in the control group from 44% to 72%. In addition, the Buteyko group had significantly reduced their ICS therapy compared with the control group ($P = .02$). None of the other differences between the groups at 6 mo were significant.	Six months after completion of the interventions, a large majority of subjects in each group displayed control of their asthma with the additional benefit of reduction in ICS use in the Buteyko group. The Buteyko technique or an intensive program delivered by a chest physiotherapist appear to provide additional benefit for adult patients with asthma who are being treated with ICS.	Adults; Buteyko (mind-body)

(continued on next page)

Table 2
(continued)

Authors, Primary	Design	Population	Results	Conclusions	Categories/Domain
Freidin and Timmermans,[28] 2008	Qualitative, open-ended individual interviews	50 mothers of children with asthma	The experience with biomedical treatments, social influence in mother's network of care, concerns about adverse and long-term effects of prescription asthma medicines, health care providers' responsiveness to such concerns, and familiarity with alternative treatments explain why some families rely on alternative medicine and others do not.	Rather than constituting vastly different demographic user profiles or reflecting diverging health beliefs, the incorporation of alternative treatments in asthma care follows a decision-making process in which experiences with prescribed drugs are socially validated and evaluated.	Children; various CAM modalities
Sidora-Arcoleo et al,[107] 2008	Qualitative, structured individual interviews	228 parents of 5- to 12-y-old children with asthma	Seventy-one percent of parents reported using CAM and/or over-the-counter medication for children's asthma management, and 54% of those parents did not disclose usage. Seventy-five percent "did not think" to discuss it. Better parent-health care provider relationship led to increased disclosure.	Health care providers can play an important role in creating an environment where parents feel comfortable sharing information about their children's asthma management strategies in order to arrive at a shared asthma management plan for the child, leading to improved asthma health outcomes.	Children; various CAM modalities

Mehl-Madrona et al,[25] 2007	Randomized controlled trial	89 individuals with asthma were randomly assignment to 1 of 5 groups: acupuncture, craniosacral therapy, acupuncture and craniosacral, attention control, and waiting list control	When treatment was compared with the control group, statistically treatment was significantly better than the control group in improving asthma quality of life, whereas reducing medication use with pulmonary function test results remained the same. However, the combination of acupuncture and craniosacral treatment was not superior to each therapy alone. In fact, although all active patients received 12 treatment sessions, those who received all treatments from one practitioner had statistically significant reductions in anxiety when compared with those receiving the same number of treatments from multiple practitioners. No effects on depression were found.	Acupuncture and/or craniosacral therapy are potentially useful adjuncts to the conventional care of adults with asthma, but the combination of the two does not provide additional benefit over each therapy alone.	Adults; acupuncture (mind-body); craniosacral therapy (manipulative and body-based practices)

(continued on next page)

Table 2
(continued)

Authors, Primary	Design	Population	Results	Conclusions	Categories/Domain
Sawni and Thomas,[106] 2007	Survey, descriptive	648 pediatricians responded to the survey	More than 96% of pediatricians responding believed their patients were using CAM. Discussions of CAM use were initiated by the family (70%) and only 37% of pediatricians asked about CAM use as part of routine medical history. Most (84%) said more CME courses should be offered on CAM and 71% said they would consider referring patients to CAM practitioners. Medical conditions referred for CAM included chronic problems (headaches, pain management,	Pediatricians have a positive attitude toward CAM. Most believe that their patients are using CAM, that asking about CAM should be part of routine medical history, would consider referring to a CAM practitioner and want more education on CAM.	Pediatricians; various CAM modalities

| | | | asthma, backaches) (86%), diseases with no known cure (55.5%) or failure of conventional therapies (56%), behavioral problems (49%), and psychiatric disorders (47%). American-born, US medical school graduates, general pediatricians, and pediatricians who ask/talk about CAM were most likely to believe their patients used CAM ($P<.01$). | Health care providers who educate themselves on CAM therapies that parents use for asthma can then discuss the implications of using these therapies and potentially improve adherence to the prescribed medication regimen. | Children; various CAM modalities |
| Sidora-Arcoleo et al,[34] 2007 | Survey, correlational | 228 parents and their 5 to12-y-old children with asthma | 65% of parents reported using CAM. Usage was highest among black, poor, less educated parents and children with persistent symptoms. Types of CAM differed by poverty and a trend for differences by race and education emerged. | | |

(continued on next page)

Table 2
(continued)

Authors, Primary	Design	Population	Results	Conclusions	Categories/Domain
George et al,[29] 2006	Qualitative, in-depth interviews	28 individuals who self-identified as being African Americans, low income, and an inner-city resident	Sixty-four percent of participants held biologically correct causal models of asthma, although 100% reported the use of at least 1 CAM for asthma. Biologically based therapies, humoral balance, and prayer were the most popular CAM. Although most subjects trusted prescription asthma medicine, there was a preference for integration of CAM with conventional asthma treatment. CAM was considered natural, effective, and potentially curative. Sixty-three percent of participants reported nonadherence to conventional therapies in the 2 wk before the research interview. Neither CAM nor nonmedical causal models altered most individuals' (93%) willingness to use prescription	Clinicians should be aware of patient-generated causal models of asthma and use of CAM in this population. Discussing patients' desire for an integrated approach to asthma management and involving social networks are 2 strategies that may enhance patient provider partnerships and treatment fidelity.	Adults; various CAM modalities

medication. Three possibly dangerous CAM were identified.

Mickleborough et al,[52] 2006	Randomized controlled trial	16 asthmatic patients with documented exercise-induced bronchoconstriction participated in the study	On the normal and placebo diet, subjects exhibited EIB; however, the fish oil diet improved pulmonary function to below the diagnostic exercise-induced bronchoconstriction threshold, with a concurrent reduction in bronchodilator use. Induced sputum differential cell count percentage and concentrations of LTC 4-LTE4, PGD2, IL-1, and TNF were significantly reduced before and following exercise on the fish oil diet compared with the normal and placebo diets. There was a significant reduction in LTB4 and a significant increase in LTB5 generation from activated PMNLs on the fish oil diet compared to the normal and placebo diets.	Data suggest that fish oil supplementation may represent a potentially beneficial nonpharmacologic intervention for exercise-induced bronchoconstriction.	Adults; fish oil (natural products)

(continued on next page)

Table 2
(continued)

Authors, Primary	Design	Population	Results	Conclusions	Categories/Domain
Nahin et al,[45] 2006	Survey, descriptive	3072 ambulatory individuals aged 75 and older	In logistic regression models, multivitamin use was associated with female sex, a higher income, a higher modified Mini-Mental State Examination score, difficulty with mobility, and asthma history; use of any other vitamin or mineral was associated with female sex, white race, nonsmoking, more years of schooling, difficulty walking, a history of osteoporosis, and reading health and senior magazines.	There were substantial differences between individuals who used vitamins and minerals and those who used NVNMDS. These data require that trial investigators pay close attention to participant use of off-protocol dietary supplements. In addition, these findings may help identify elderly individuals likely to combine nonvitamin/nonmineral dietary supplement and prescription drugs.	Older adults; nonvitamin/nonmineral dietary supplement (natural products)

| Aboussafy et al,[82] 2005 | Intervention trial | 31 adults with asthma participated in the study | The cold pressor test, asthma interview, and progressive muscle relaxation produced significant decreases in airflow compared with the baseline period. The cold pressor test and progressive muscle relaxation produced significant, complementary increases in vagal tone. | These results suggest that passive coping stressors and other stimuli (eg, certain forms of relaxation) that elicit increased vagal tone may be associated with poorer asthma control, a view consistent with a significant negative correlation between the participant's mean vagal tone response to the tasks and score on a measure of asthma self-efficacy. | Adults; progressive muscle relaxation (mind-body) |

(continued on next page)

Table 2
(continued)

Authors, Primary	Design	Population	Results	Conclusions	Categories/Domain
Ang et al,[36] 2005	Survey, correlational	152 subjects were interviewed on the use of CAM for their children.	Compared with parents of the healthy and asthma groups, parents of the HIV group were less likely to be employed, were less likely to have private insurance, were less likely to have a high school or college education, and were more likely to be black. Interestingly, 38% of the healthy children parents used CAM in their children compared with 22% in the HIV group and 25% in the asthma group. More than 80% of all three groups paid out of pocket for their use of CAM in their	This study revealed a relatively high rate of CAM usage by parents of all three study groups. Although parents of children with HIV infection were more likely to want CAM as part of their children's medical care, their rate of CAM usage was not higher than that in well children. This may be related to their socioeconomic factors. A larger and more diverse study population may provide more information on factors contributing to CAM usage in chronically ill and well children.	Children; various CAM modalities

			children. Within these groups, HIV parents were more likely to want CAM as part of their child's medical care and were more likely to believe that CAM was expensive.	
Dobson et al,[66] 2005	Intervention trial	4 children participants	Results demonstrated that relaxation and guided imagery significantly improved the lung functioning of 3 of 4 participants in the study. Furthermore, overall happiness improved for 1 participant in the study, state anxiety decreased for 2 of the 4 participants, and trait anxiety decreased for all 4 participants.	Relaxation and guided imagery were found to be effective in improving the lung functioning of 3 of the 4 study participants included. Children; relaxation and guided imagery (mind-body)

(continued on next page)

Table 2
(continued)

Authors, Primary	Design	Population	Results	Conclusions	Categories/Domain
Klein et al,[104] 2005	Qualitative, focus groups	81 adolescents: suburban adolescents, urban minority adolescents, adolescents with chronic illness, (asthma, eating disorders, and diabetes), and patients of complementary/ alternative practitioners in Monroe County, NY	Most adolescents are familiar with "herbal medicine," "herbal remedies," or "nutritional supplements," and are able to name specific products or CAM therapies; however, many are unfamiliar with the term "alternative medicine." Adolescents are more familiar with remedies or CAM therapies commonly used by people from their own cultural or ethnic background. Older	Most adolescents are familiar with culturally based herbal products and nutritional supplements, used for treatment of illnesses, and not for preventive care. Providers and researchers should consider chronic illness status and culture/ family tradition, and clarify terms, when asking adolescents about self-care, over-the-counter, or CAM.	Children; various CAM modalities (natural products)

suburban females and those with chronic illnesses are more familiar with herbs and supplements than other adolescents. Most supplement use is conceptually linked with treating illness rather than with preventive care.

| Sabina et al,[26] 2005 | Randomized controlled trial (pilot) | 62 participants with asthma | Intention-to-treat analysis was performed. Significant within-group differences in post bronchodilator FEV(1) and morning symptom scores were apparent in both groups at 4 and 16 wk; however, no significant differences between groups were observed on any outcome measures. | Iyengar yoga conferred no appreciable benefit in mild-to-moderate asthma. Circumstances under which yoga is of benefit in asthma management, if any, remain to be determined. | Adults; Yoga (mind-body) |

(continued on next page)

Table 2
(continued)

Authors, Primary	Design	Population	Results	Conclusions	Categories/Domain
Epstein et al,[75] 2004	Randomized controlled trial (pilot)	68 adults with symptomatic asthma	There was little evidence of statistical change in this feasibility study; yet, valuable lessons were learned. Paired t tests indicated there was a significant difference in the total power scores in the imagery group, and in the expected direction and the choices subscale of the power instrument from weeks 1 to 16 of the study. Eight (47%) of 17 participants in the mental imagery group reduced or	Findings related to major outcome measures must be viewed with caution because of the small sample size resulting from attrition related to labor intensiveness and, therefore, low statistical power. However, the study did provide significant data to plan a larger scale study of the use of mental imagery with adults with asthma. The study also demonstrated that imagery is inexpensive,	Adults; mental imagery (mind-body)

discontinued their medications. Three of 16 (19%) participants in the control group reduced their medications; none discontinued. Chi-square indicated differences between groups. Persons who reduced or discontinued their medications showed neither an increase in pulmonary function before medication discontinuation, nor a fall in these parameters following discontinuation.

safe and, with training, can be used as an adjunct therapy by patients themselves. Its efficacy needs additional exploration. Further research for adults with asthma who practice imagery is important, as current treatments are not entirely efficacious. Lessons learned in this study may facilitate improvement in research designs.

(continued on next page)

Table 2
(continued)

Authors, Primary	Design	Population	Results	Conclusions	Categories/Domain
Handelman et al,[43] 2004	Qualitative, explanatory models	19 children with 17 mothers from a variety of cultural backgrounds were interviewed	Among children, contagion was the primary explanatory model for asthma etiology (53%). Twenty-five percent of children reported fear of dying from asthma, whereas fear of their child dying from asthma was reported by 76% of mothers. Mothers reported a variety of explanatory models, some culturally specific, but most reported biomedical concepts of etiology, pathophysiology, and triggers. Although 76% of mothers knew the	The traditional focus of asthma education is not sufficient to ensure adherence. Asthma education for children should address their views of etiology and fears about dying from asthma. Conversations with parents about their explanatory models and beliefs about medications and alternative therapies could assist in understanding and responding to parental concerns and choices about medications and help achieve better adherence.	Children; various CAM modalities

names of more than one of their children's medications, 47% thought their child's medications all had similar functions. Thirty-five percent of families used herbal treatments and 35% incorporated religion into asthma treatment. Seventy-one percent of families had discontinued medications and 23% reported currently not giving anti-inflammatory medication. Reasons for discontinuing daily medications included fears of unknown side effects (53%), addiction (18%), tachyphylaxis (18%), and feeling that their child was being given too much medicine (23%).

(continued on next page)

Table 2
(continued)

Authors, Primary	Design	Population	Results	Conclusions	Categories/Domain
Lehrer et al,[27] 2004	Randomized controlled trial	94 adult outpatient volunteers with asthma	Compared with the 2 control groups, subjects in both of the 2 heart rate variability biofeedback groups were prescribed less medication, with minimal differences between the 2 active treatments. Improvements averaged 1 full level of asthma severity. Measures from forced oscillation pneumography similarly showed improvement in pulmonary function. A placebo effect influenced an improvement in asthma symptoms, but not in pulmonary function. Groups did not differ in the occurrence of severe asthma flares.	The results suggest that heart rate variability biofeedback may prove to be a useful adjunct to asthma treatment and may help to reduce dependence on steroid medications. Further evaluation of this method is warranted.	Adults; biofeedback (mind-body)
Milner et al,[42] 2004	Survey, correlational (longitudinal cohort survey study)	There were 8000 total patients in the study. The cohort data were taken from the National Center for Health Statistics 1988 National Maternal-	The overall incidence of asthma was 10.5% and of food allergy was 4.9%. In univariate analysis, male gender, smoker in the household, child care,	Early vitamin supplementation is associated with increased risk for asthma in black children and food allergies in exclusively	Children; Vitamins (natural products)

Infant Health Survey, which followed pregnant women and their newborns, and the 1991 Longitudinal Follow-up of the same patients.

prematurity (<37 wk), being black, no history of breastfeeding, lower income, and lower education were associated with higher risk for asthma. Child care, higher levels of education, income, and history of breastfeeding were associated with a higher risk for food allergies. In multivariate logistic analyses, a history of vitamin use within the first 6 mo of life was associated with a higher risk for asthma in black infants (OR: 1.27). Early vitamin use was also associated with a higher risk for food allergies in the exclusively formula-fed population (OR: 1.63). Vitamin use at 3 y of age was associated with increased risk for food allergies but not asthma in both breastfed (OR: 1.62; 95% CI: 1.19–2.21) and exclusively formula-fed infants (OR: 1.39; 95% CI: 1.03–1.88).

formula-fed children. Additional study is warranted to examine which components most strongly contribute to this risk.

(continued on next page)

Table 2
(continued)

Authors, Primary	Design	Population	Results	Conclusions	Categories/Domain
Lanski et al,[44] 2003	Survey, descriptive	142 families participated in the study	Forty-five percent of caregivers reported giving their child an herbal product, and 88% of these caregivers had at least 1 y of college education. Of the children receiving these therapies, 53% had been given 1 type and 27% were given 3 or more in the past year. The most common therapies reportedly used were aloe plant/juice (44%), *Echinacea* (33%), and sweet oil (25%). The most dangerous potential herbal and prescription medication combination reported was ephedra and albuterol in an adolescent with asthma. The most unusual products reportedly used included turpentine, pine needles, and cowchips. Of all people	Herbal and home therapies are commonly used in this pediatric population. An unexpectedly wide variety of products were reportedly given to this patient population. Caregivers reported limited knowledge regarding potential adverse medication interactions and side effects. Limited discussions with the child's primary health care provider were reported. It is therefore important for health care providers to have knowledge about herbal medications, to inquire about their use, and to educate families about the risk/benefit as well as potential interactions these products may have with over-the-counter and prescription medications.	Children; Herbs (natural products)

			interviewed, 77% did not believe or were uncertain if herbal products had any side effects and only 27% could name a potential side effect. Sixty-six percent were unsure or thought that herbal products did not interact with other medications and only 2 people correctly named a drug interaction. Of the people who used these therapies, 80% reported either friends or relatives as their primary source of information. Only 45% of those giving their children herbal products report discussing the use with their child's primary health care provider.		
Peck et al,[67] 2003	Intervention trial	4 children with asthma	With the introduction of the intervention, it was found that FEV(1) improved and anxiety decreased in all students. FEF25–75 improved in 3 of the 4 participants.	Relaxation and guided imagery improved asthma outcomes	Children; relaxation and guided imagery (mind-body)

(continued on next page)

Table 2
(continued)

Authors, Primary	Design	Population	Results	Conclusions	Categories/Domain
Anbar,[69] 2002	Intervention trial	303 patients with pulmonary symptoms attributable to psychological issues, discomfort due to medications, or fear of procedures	Hypnotherapy was associated with improvement in 80% of patients with persistent asthma, chest pain/ pressure, habit cough, hyperventilation, shortness of breath, sighing, and vocal cord dysfunction. When improvement was reported, in some cases symptoms resolved immediately after hypnotherapy was first used. For the others, improvement was achieved after hypnosis was used for a few weeks. No patients' symptoms worsened and no new symptoms emerged following hypnotherapy.	Patients described in this report were unlikely to have achieved rapid improvement in their symptoms without the use of hypnotherapy. Therefore, hypnotherapy can be an important complementary therapy for patients in a pediatric practice.	Children; hypnosis (mind-body)
Baldwin et al,[38] 2002	Survey, correlational	508 military veterans randomly selected from Southern Arizona Veterans	Of the 508 subjects, 252 (49.6%) reported CAM use. Military veteran CAM users were	Ethnicity, education, income, and several chronic health complaints are	Adults; various CAM modalities

Administration Health Care System (Tucson) primary care patient lists

significantly more likely to be non-Hispanic white, earn more than $50 000 per year (both $P<.05$), and have more than 12 y of education ($P<.01$). Current high daily stress, perceived negative impact of military life on physical or mental health, and physician-diagnosed chronic illnesses (eg, gastrointestinal problems, insomnia, and asthma) were statistically associated with CAM use. Regression analysis provided adjusted odds ratios and indicated that ethnicity (non-Hispanic white), higher education, greater current daily stress, and overseas military experience were significant predictors of CAM use by these veterans (each $P<.05$).

consistent with civilian CAM use. Findings also suggest, however, that physicians providing conventional medical care need to be aware of experiences unique to CAM-using military veterans.

(continued on next page)

Table 2
(continued)

Authors, Primary	Design	Population	Results	Conclusions	Categories/Domain
Hockemeyer and Smyth,[78] 2002	Randomized controlled trial (between-groups, prospective experimental design)	60 college students with asthma	The treatment group showed significant improvement in measures of lung function compared with the placebo group, but analysis revealed no differences in measures of perceived stress.	These findings provide initial support for the feasibility of self-administered manual-based interventions and some evidence that they can produce health benefits in individuals with asthma and, perhaps, other chronic conditions.	Adults, relaxation, cognitive-behavioral treatment (mind-body)
Reznik et al,[30] 2002	Survey, correlational	200 children with asthma	Overall, 80% of participants reported using CAM for asthma. The most commonly reported CAM included rubs (74%), herbal teas (39%), prayer (37%), massage (36%), and Jarabe 7 syrup (24%).	Most adolescents with asthma in this study used CAM. The prevalence of CAM use in this study population was twice the national average for adults.	Children; various CAM modalities

| | | | Subjects with daily or weekly symptoms were more likely to use CAM for each episode of asthma (72% vs 51%; $P = .005$). The 61% of subjects who had a family member who used CAM were more likely to use CAM again (84% vs 39%; $P<.001$). Of the respondents, 59% reported that CAM was effective. | | |
| Wade,[72] 2002 | Intervention trial | 9 children with asthma | Results indicate that the participants showed an increase or maintenance of lung functioning after singing, whereas results were not consistent following the relaxation condition. | Singing might have a positive effect on children with asthma. | Children; music therapy; relaxation (mind-body) |

(continued on next page)

Table 2
(continued)

Authors, Primary	Design	Population	Results	Conclusions	Categories/Domain
Blanc et al,[48] 2001	Survey, correlational	300 adults with self-report of a physician diagnosis of asthma (n = 125) or rhinosinusitis without concomitant asthma (n = 175).	Any alternative practice was reported by 127 subjects (42%; 95% CI, 36%–48%). Of these, 33 subjects (26%; 95% CI, 21%–31%) were not current prescription medication users. Herbal use was reported by 72 subjects (24%), caffeine treatment by 54	Alternative treatments are frequent among adults with asthma or rhinosinusitis and should be taken into account by health-care providers and public health and policy analysts.	Adult; various CAM modalities

subjects (18%), and other alternative treatments by 66 subjects (22%). Taking into account demographic variables, subjects with asthma were more likely than those with rhinitis alone to report caffeine self-treatment for their condition (OR, 2.5; 95% CI, 1.4%–4.8%), but herbal use and other alternative treatments did not differ significantly by condition group.

(continued on next page)

Table 2
(continued)

Authors, Primary	Design	Population	Results	Conclusions	Categories/Domain
Bronfort et al,[93] 2001	Feasibility study of conducting a full-scale, randomized clinical trial	36 patients aged 6–17 y with mild and moderate persistent asthma were admitted to the study.	It is possible to blind the participants to the nature of the spinal manipulative therapy intervention, and a full-scale trial with the described design is feasible to conduct. At the end of the 12-wk intervention phase, objective lung function tests and patient-rated day and nighttime symptoms based on diary recordings showed little or no change. Of the patient-rated measures, a reduction of approximately 20% in beta(2) bronchodilator use was seen ($P = .10$). The quality-of-life scores improved by 10%–28% ($P <.01$), with	After 3 mo of combining chiropractic spinal manipulative therapy with optimal medical management for pediatric asthma, the children rated their quality of life substantially higher and their asthma severity substantially lower. These improvements were maintained at the 1-y follow-up assessment. There were no important changes in lung function or hyperresponsiveness at any time. The observed improvements are unlikely as a result of the specific effects of chiropractic spinal manipulative therapy	Children; spinal manipulation (manipulative and body-based practices)

the activity scale showing the most change. Asthma severity ratings showed a reduction of 39% ($P<.001$), and there was an overall improvement rating corresponding to 50%–75%. The pulmonologist-rated improvement was small. Similarly, the improvements in parent-rated or guardian-rated outcomes were mostly small and not statistically significant. The changes in patient-rated severity and the improvement rating remained unchanged at 12-mo posttreatment follow-up as assessed by a brief postal questionnaire.

alone, but other aspects of the clinical encounter that should not be dismissed readily. Further research is needed to assess which components of the chiropractic encounter are responsible for important improvements in patient-oriented outcomes so that they may be incorporated into the care of all patients with asthma.

(continued on next page)

Table 2
(continued)

Authors, Primary	Design	Population	Results	Conclusions	Categories/Domain
Loera et al,[19] 2001	Survey, correlational	2734 responses from the Hispanic Established Populations for the Epidemiologic Study of the Elderly (Hispanic-EPESE) 1993–1994 were analyzed	The use of herbal medicine in the 2 wk before the interview was reported by 9.8% of the sample. Chamomile and mint were the 2 most commonly used herbs. Users of herbal medicines were more likely to be women, born in Mexico, older than 75, living alone, and experiencing some financial strain. Having arthritis, urinary incontinence, asthma,	Herbal medication use is common among older Mexican Americans, particularly among those with chronic medical conditions, those who experience financial strain, and those who are very frequent users of formal health care services.	Adults; herbs (natural products)

and hip fracture were also associated with an elevated use of herbal medicines, whereas heart attacks were not. Herbal medicine use was substantially higher among individuals reporting any disability in activities of daily living, poor self-reported health, and depressive symptoms. Herbal medicine use was associated with the use of over-the-counter medications but not with prescription medications. Herbal medicine use was particularly high among respondents who had more than 24 physician visits during the year before the interview.

(continued on next page)

Table 2
(continued)

Authors, Primary	Design	Population	Results	Conclusions	Categories/Domain
Ottolini et al,[31] 2001	Survey, cross-sectional	348 parents of children completed surveys.	Forty percent (138) of parents were CAM users themselves, whereas 21% (72) had treated their child with CAM over the past year. Factors positively associated with child CAM use included parents' use of CAM ($P<.0001$); greater parent age ($P = .0005$); greater child age ($P = .001$); and complaints of frequent respiratory illnesses, asthma, headaches, and nosebleeds. Ethnicity and parental education were not associated with child CAM use. More than 50% of pediatric CAM users reported specific vitamin supplementation, whereas 25% used other nutritional supplements or elimination diets, and more than 40% used	Treatment of children with CAM is common and is frequently undertaken by parents without the knowledge or advice of their pediatrician.	Children; various CAM modalities

			herbal therapies. Thirty-two percent of CAM users had visited a CAM practitioner; 81% of pediatric CAM users would have liked to discuss it with their pediatrician, but only 36% did so.		
Smyth et al,[74] 2001	Intervention trial	20 adults with asthma	Relaxation training was successful, but did not lead to the hypothesized reduction in overall cortisol levels. Participants using corticosteroid medication showed increases in cortisol after relaxation, whereas those not using corticosteroids showed decreases in cortisol ($P<.05$). Relaxation altered the cortisol reactivity to stress ($P = .007$); before relaxation training, cortisol levels increased after a stressor, whereas following relaxation training, cortisol levels decreased after a stressor.	This study suggests that relaxation training can influence cortisol secretion in individuals with asthma, but that these effects differ from those observed in healthy individuals and may be influenced by corticosteroid medication use.	Adults; breathing relaxation (mind-body)

(continued on next page)

Table 2
(continued)

Authors, Primary	Design	Population	Results	Conclusions	Categories/Domain
Hailemaskel et al,[46] 2001	Survey, descriptive	100 prospective adult customers visiting a health food store during a consecutive 5-day period completed a 20-item questionnaire	The 4 most common diseases reported were allergies, high blood pressure, depression, and asthma. The top 4 herbals used were St John's Wort, *Echinacea*, ginseng, and golden seal. Results identified 6 *cases* with potential herbal-drug interactions, 5 *cases* with potential herb-disease interactions, and 19% with potential adverse drug reactions.	The data from this survey suggest that although the use of herbals is widespread and commonly accepted, it is necessary to educate consumers about the potential risks involved in such unmonitored use.	Adults; herbs (natural products)
Smyth et al,[73] 1999	Intervention trial (pilot)	22 community residents with asthma	Listening to a 20-min audiotaped relaxation training program led to decreased negative mood and stressor report, but was unrelated to positive mood. The report of asthma symptoms decreased over time following relaxation training, and peak expiratory flow rate was significantly increased by relaxation training.	This study provides evidence that a brief, inexpensive, tape-recorded relaxation intervention can improve well-being, decrease symptom report, and improve peak expiratory flow rate in asthma. The relatively inexpensive and low-risk nature of the treatment, as well as its benefit to quality of life, support its utility as a supplemental treatment.	Adults; breathing relaxation (mind-body)

| Balon et al,[94] 1998 | Randomized controlled trial | 91 children who had continuing symptoms of asthma despite usual medical therapy | Eighty children (38 in the active-treatment group and 42 in the simulated-treatment group) had outcome data that could be evaluated. There were small increases (7–12 L per minute) in peak expiratory flow in the morning and the evening in both treatment groups, with no significant differences between the groups in the degree of change from base line (morning peak expiratory flow, $P = .49$ at 2 months and $P = .82$ at 4 months). Symptoms of asthma and use of 3-agonists decreased and the quality of life increased in both groups, with no significant differences between the groups. There were no significant changes in spirometric measurements or airway responsiveness. | In children with mild or moderate asthma, the addition of chiropractic spinal manipulation to usual medical care provided no benefit. | Children; spinal manipulation (manipulative and body-based practices) |

(continued on next page)

Table 2
(continued)

Authors, Primary	Design	Population	Results	Conclusions	Categories/Domain
Davis et al,[108] 1998	Survey, correlational	564 participants have completed the study surveys	The survey population was 46% male and 43% female; 11% did not specify gender. They ranged in age from younger than 31 y to older than 70. The largest group (37%) of respondents held degrees as medical doctors, 27% held doctorates in CAM-related disciplines, 11% had registered nursing degrees, 4% were acupuncturists, and 18% did not specify their training. Practice characteristics between MD and non-MD asthma care providers did not differ. Most had general practices (75%) seeing all ages of patients. MDs were less likely to use CAM techniques for asthma	The predominance of diet and nutrition supplementation used by MDs and non-MDs suggests that further attention and research efforts should be directed toward this area of CAM practice. Other CAM practices, such as botanicals, meditation, and homeopathy appear to warrant research efforts. Differences between MDs and non-MDs in their use of such therapies may reflect different philosophies as well as training.	Adults; various CAM modalities

compared with non-MDs. Both groups identified dietary and nutritional approaches as their most prevalent and useful asthma treatment option. Use of botanicals, meditation, and homeopathy were frequently cited; statistically significant differences appeared in the rankings of treatment usefulness and prevalence between MDs and non-MDs. Non-MD asthma care providers were more likely to ask patients about their use of CAM treatments for asthma than MDs (92% vs 70%), whereas both groups showed statistically significant increases in their levels of patient inquiries compared with 2 y previously (up 9% and 8% for MDs and non-MDs respectively).

(continued on next page)

Table 2
(continued)

Authors, Primary	Design	Population	Results	Conclusions	Categories/Domain
Field et al,[92] 1998	Randomized controlled trial	32 children with asthma	The younger children who received massage therapy showed an immediate decrease in behavioral anxiety and cortisol levels after massage. Also, their attitude toward asthma and their peak air flow and other pulmonary functions improved over the course of the study. The older children who received massage therapy reported lower anxiety after the massage. Their attitude toward asthma also improved over the study, but only one measure of pulmonary function (FEF 25%–75%) improved.	The reason for the smaller therapeutic benefit in the older children is unknown; however, it appears that daily massage improves airway caliber and control of asthma.	Children; massage (manipulative and body-based practices); relaxation (mind body)
Vedanthan et al,[76] 1998	Randomized controlled trial	17 adults with asthma	Analysis of the data showed that the subjects in the yoga group reported a significant degree of	Yoga techniques seem beneficial as an adjunct to the medical management of asthma.	Adults; yoga (mind-body)

			relaxation, positive attitude, and better yoga exercise tolerance. There was also a tendency toward lesser usage of beta adrenergic inhalers. The pulmonary functions did not vary significantly between yoga and control groups.		
Blanc et al,[49] 1997	Survey, correlational	601 adults with asthma recruited from a random sample of pulmonary and allergy specialists.	Herbal asthma self-treatment was reported by 46 (8%); coffee or black tea self-treatment by 36 (6%), epinephrine or ephedrine OTC use by 36 (6%), and any of the 3 practices by 98 subjects (16%). Adjusting for demographic and illness covariates, herbal use (OR 2.5) and coffee or black tea use (OR 3.1) were associated with asthma hospitalization; OTC use was not (OR 0.8).	Even among adults with access to specialty care for asthma, self-treatment with nonprescription products was common and was associated with increased risk of reported hospitalization. This association does not appear to be accounted for by illness severity or other disease covariates. It may reflect delay in utilization of more efficacious treatments.	Adults; herbs (natural products)

(continued on next page)

Table 2
(continued)

Authors, Primary	Design	Population	Results	Conclusions	Categories/Domain
Kohen and Wynne,[70] 1997	Intervention trial	25 children with asthma and their parent(s)	Following participation in the Preschool Asthma Program, physician visits for asthma were reduced ($P = .0013$) and parents reported increased confidence in self-management skills. Symptom severity scores improved significantly after participation ($P<.001$). A possible association was noted between participation in the program and parental expectations or projections of future outcome ($.05<P<.1$). No changes were observed in the frequency of asthma episodes or in pulmonary function tests before and after the program.	With the hypnotherapeutic approach of imagery, preschoolers developed new cooperation in asthma-care skills, including cooperative and consistent performance of peak flow measurements.	Children; hypnosis (mind-body)
Lehrer et al,[83] 1997	Intervention trial	87 adults with asthma	Changes in forced expiratory volume/forced vital capacity were negatively correlated with those in cardiac interbeat interval. Contrary to	Results suggest that the immediate effects of generalized relaxation instruction can be associated with a parasympathetic rebound, which, in	Adults; progressive muscle relaxation (mind-body)

the theory of a vagal-trigeminal reflex as mediator for relaxation-induced improvement in asthma, decreases in pulmonary function occurred during relaxation sessions, accompanied by increases in cardiovagal activity, and within-session changes in frontal EMG in the 1st session of training were positively associated with changes in forced expiratory volume/forced vital capacity. However, consistent with this hypothesis, first-session frontalis EMG changes were positively associated with changes in respiratory sinus arrhythmia, and last-session changes in cardiac interbeat interval were positively associated with changes in forced expiratory volume/forced vital capacity.

turn, may induce countertherapeutic changes in asthma.

(continued on next page)

Table 2
(continued)

Authors, Primary	Design	Population	Results	Conclusions	Categories/Domain
Coen et al,[68] 1996	Randomized controlled (pilot) study	20 participants, aged 12–22 y, with nonsteroid-dependent reactive airway disease participated.	Results showed decreased asthma severity and decreased facial muscle tension in the experimental group but not in the control group. Improvements in asthma severity were correlated with decreases in facial muscle tension. No effects on pulmonary function were seen. Data on immune measures revealed significant decreases in immunoglobulins in both groups related to seasonal change. Increases in CD4 and CD8 lymphocyte counts were observed more frequently in the experimental group than in the controls.	The findings suggest that biofeedback-assisted relaxation training has potential for improvement of asthma severity and immune function in young individuals with asthma.	Children; adults; biofeedback-assisted relaxation (mind-body)
Lehrer et al,[84] 1994	Randomized controlled trial	106 medically prestabilized adults with asthma	Relaxation-group subjects reported feeling the most deeply relaxed and produced the greatest improvement in FEF during the last presession assessment	Listening to music produced greater decreases in peaks of tension than progressive muscle relaxation, and it produced greater compliance with	Adults; music therapy; progressive muscle relaxation (mind-body)

Source	Design	Subjects	Results	Conclusion	Category
			period. All groups evidenced decreases in asthma symptoms. All groups showed decreases in pulmonary function immediately after relaxation sessions. None of the changes in pulmonary function reached levels that are accepted in drug trials to be of clinical significance, and the therapeutic changes occurred only in the situation where training was rendered.	relaxation practice, but it did not produce any specific therapeutic effects on asthma.	
Kotses et al,[64] 1991	Randomized controlled trial	29 children with asthma	As compared with the facial stability subjects, the facial relaxation subjects exhibited higher pulmonary scores, more positive attitudes toward asthma, and lower chronic anxiety during the follow-up period. Subjects in the 2 groups, however, did not differ on self-rated asthma severity, medication usage, frequency of asthma attacks, or self-concept.	Based on the improvements we observed in pulmonary, attitude, and anxiety measures, we concluded that biofeedback training for facial relaxation contributes to the self-control of asthma and would be a valuable addition to asthma self-management programs.	Children; biofeedback-assisted relaxation (mind-body)

(continued on next page)

Table 2
(continued)

Authors, Primary	Design	Population	Results	Conclusions	Categories/Domain
Murphy et al,[120] 1989	Survey, correlational	12 adults with asthma	Hypnotic susceptibility measures appeared to be related to several measures of improvement in asthma symptoms, and this relationship was similar in both relaxation and placebo treatments.	Findings indicate that hypnotic susceptibility and suggestive processes play similar roles in both interventions and that hypnotic susceptibility may be a useful predictor of response to psychological treatment in asthma.	Adults; hypnosis (mind-body)
Tashkin et al,[81] 1985	Randomized controlled	25 patients with moderate to severe asthma	Two-way analysis of variance failed to reveal a significant effect of either form of acupuncture on symptoms, medication use, or lung function measurements. Similarly, no significant acute effect of acupuncture on lung function, self-ratings of efficacy, or physician's physical findings was found by covariance analysis or the	The findings failed to demonstrate any short-term or long-term benefit of acupuncture therapy in the management of moderate to severe asthma.	Adults; acupuncture (mind-body)

Alexander et al,[61] 1979	Intervention trial	14 children with chronic and severe asthma	Wilcoxon signed-rank test. When data during the entire course of the study were examined on an individual basis by analysis of variance with repeated measures, only two subjects demonstrated significantly favorable responses to real vs placebo acupuncture, but one subject demonstrated the reverse, suggesting that these responses were not specifically related to acupuncture therapy.	Children; relaxation (mind-body)
			Heart rate, and to some extent, muscle tension results confirm the attainment of relaxed states. However, the lung function results fail to substantiate the previous, preliminary findings of a clinically meaningful change in pulmonary function following relaxation.	Relaxation did not have significant effect on lung function

(continued on next page)

Table 2
(continued)

Authors, Primary	Design	Population	Results	Conclusions	Categories/Domain
Wilson et al,[77] 1975	Intervention trial	21 adults with asthma	As compared with the initial values recorded before intervention, significant improvement in forced expiratory volume, peak expiratory flow rate, and airway resistance was noted.	The results indicated that transcendental meditation is a useful adjunct in treating asthma.	Adults; meditation (mind-body)
Alexander et al,[62] 1972	Randomized controlled trial	44 children with asthma	Results show that relaxation subjects manifested a significant mean increase in peak expiratory flow rate over sessions, compared with a nonsignificant mean peak expiratory flow decrease for controls.	Relaxation was effective to increase the peak expiratory flow rate.	Children; relaxation (mind-body)

Abbreviations: ACQ, Asthma Control Questionnaire; AQLQ, Asthma Quality of Life Questionnaire; BMI, body mass index; CAM, complementary and alternative medicine; EIB, Exercise induced bronchoconstriction; EMG, electromyogram; FEF, forced expiratory flow; FEV(1), forced expiratory volume in 1 second; HCP, health care provider; IL, interleukin; LTB, Leukotriene B4 and B5; OTC, over the counter; PC 20, provocative concentration of a substance (methacholine) causing a 20% fall in the Forced Expiratory Volume in 1 Second; PMNL, Polymorphonuclear Leukocyte; PR, Prevalence Ratio; TNF, tumor necrosis factor.

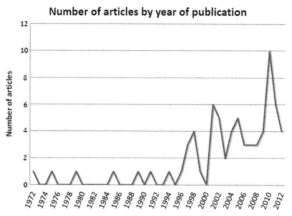

Fig. 2. Number of articles by year of publication.

qualitative research using in-depth interviews. Specifically, 42% of the reviewed articles (n = 30, see **Table 2** for details) reported results of surveys, using either descriptive or correlational designs. Most of these used secondary data from large-scale, comprehensively developed and thoroughly conducted national US surveys. For example, Joubert and colleagues[13] analyzed data from the National Health Interview Survey (NHIS), the principal source of information on the health of the civilian noninstitutionalized US population. The NHIS is one of the major US data-collection programs.[14] Using secondary NHIS data, the researchers were able to analyze 3327 responses of individuals with asthma across the United States to identify the association between asthma episodes in the past 12 months and CAM use, controlling for comorbid conditions. Several other investigators using similar survey designs were able to identify significant patterns of CAM use and its affects in the United States[15-19] and in Canada.[8,11]

Only one-third of the reviewed studies (n = 21) were RCTs despite RCTs being considered the "gold-standard" design when causal relationships between the treatments and health outcomes need to be established.[20] Further, there were several issues related to the quality of several of the RCT studies identified from this review. One example is an application of a technique that addresses the problems associated with incomplete data because of participant withdrawal, described as "intention-to-treat" analysis (ITT). In the ITT approach, all the participants are retained in study data analyses regardless of their path through the trial and completion of the study.[21,22] Participants are retained in the treatment group they are randomized to ("as randomized"), rather than being classified according to the actual treatment they received ("as treated"). In general, ITT analysis produces an unbiased estimate of treatment effectiveness.[22] One fundamental assumption of the ITT method is that missing data and participant withdrawal are not related to the unobserved outcome. ITT also assumes that compliance among those who remain in the trial and those who withdraw is equivalent. Sensitivity analysis and other statistical methods were developed to validate this assumption.[21] In our review, 24% of the RCT studies used the ITT approach in their analysis[23-27]; however, some of the researchers did not mention whether the assumptions about the missing data and adherence were validated and if sensitivity analysis was performed.[23,24] This lack of information significantly limits the interpretation of the results of the reviewed RCTs.

Thirteen of the reviewed studies (18%) were conducted using quasi-experimental designs (mostly a 1-group pretest posttest design). This type of studies is important, especially when experimental methods are impractical or unethical to use; however, it is challenging to make definitive causal inferences using results of these studies. Several statistical methods were recently developed to enhance the causality conclusions of quasi-experimental studies, for example propensity scoring that reduces the confounding effects of covariates. Unfortunately, we did not identify that these methods were used in the reviewed manuscripts. In addition, it was noted that the number of quasi-experimental studies has decreased over time, with only 2 articles using this methodology published since 2005.

The balance of the reviewed studies (10%) used qualitative methods for the data analysis. Application of qualitative methods helps researchers to glean important personal information that is usually inaccessible otherwise. For example, Freidin and Timmermans[28] used open-ended questions to understand the experience with biomedical treatments, social influences, and concerns about adverse and long-term effects of prescription asthma medicines among mothers of children with asthma. In another study, George and colleagues[29] used in-depth interviews to identify causal models of asthma and the context of conventional prescription versus CAM use in low-income African American adults with asthma. More studies using qualitative methods are needed to further understand factors related to asthma medication adherence, possible adverse effects of CAM therapies, and other issues.

Patterns of CAM Use for Asthma

High CAM prevalence rates have been reported for both children and adults with asthma. Pediatric use has been reported to be as high as 80% when folk medicine (which includes prayer) is included in the broad definition of what constitutes a CAM practice.[30] Approximately one-quarter of children reported CAM use for asthma in the past year[16,31] and use is highest in those children with poorer asthma control,[11,32] financial barriers to conventional care,[16] greater severity,[16] more symptoms,[30,33,34] or a CAM-using parent.[7,30,31,35] As much as 80% of pediatric CAM care required an out-of-pocket expenditure.[36]

Similarly, CAM use for adult asthma is extremely high (96%–100%) when survey questions include folk medicine/prayer.[29,37] More than 70% report CAM for symptom management in the past month[33] and prevalence is higher in adults with work-related asthma,[15] financial obstacles to accessing care,[17,19] more symptoms,[17,33] more stress,[38] and more frequent attacks.[13]

CAM Domains

Fig. 1 presents the reviewed articles by CAM domain. Almost half (47%) of the reviewed articles focused on multiple CAM modalities, with 30% concentrated solely on mind-body CAM approaches, 15% on natural products, and the remainder on manipulative and body-based practices (6%) or energy-field healing (2%).

Natural Products

As seen in **Table 1**, natural products encompass a wide variety of ingestible goods that include herbs, vitamins, minerals, specialized diets, dietary supplements, and botanicals. Unfortunately, much of what we know about their use is limited to prevalence surveys; few experimental studies have been conducted.

Unlike prescription drugs, manufacturers do not have to prove either the safety or the effectiveness of natural products. In fact, labels such as "safe," "standardized," "verified," or "certified" do not guarantee quality or consistency.[39] For example, herbal therapies may contain more than one herb, the wrong species of herb, a higher or lower dose of active ingredient than listed on the label, or contaminants, such as other herbs, prescription medicine, pesticides, and heavy metals.[40] In addition, natural products are not inert and may interfere with prescription drugs to cause unintended side effects.[41]

Natural Products for Pediatric Asthma

Although vitamin supplementation is commonly used for pediatric asthma,[16,31,35] a large longitudinal cohort survey study suggests that early vitamin supplementation may actually increase risk for asthma and food allergies in certain vulnerable populations.[42] High use of herbal therapies is also reported,[16,30,31,43,44] including over-the-counter (OTC) topical chest rubs made with camphor, eucalyptus oil and menthol,[30] herbal teas,[30] aloe plant juice,[44] *Echinacea*,[44] sweet oil (eg, olive, rapeseed, almond),[44] and an herbal cough syrup sold in *botanicas* containing sweet almond oil, castor oil, tolu (tree resin), wild cherry, licorice, cocillana (grape bark), and honey.[30] Atypical products reported include ephedra, turpentine, pine needles, and dried cow dung.[44]

Children with asthma also use dietary supplements,[35] nutritional supplements, and elimination diets[31] without scientific evaluation of their safety or effectiveness.[4] In one study, Covar and colleagues[24] randomized children with asthma to either a nutritional formula composed of antioxidants, omega-3 and omega-6 fatty acids, or a control formula; there were no differences in asthma-free days between groups, although inflammatory biomarkers decreased in the children receiving the nutritional formula.

Natural Products for Adult Asthma

Multivitamin use is associated with asthma in older adults[45] and herbal products are widely used (93%) by the general adult asthma population.[29,46] Commonly used herbal therapies include chamomile, mint, and *Echinacea*.[19,29,47–49] In addition, OTC ephedra products, as well as coffee and tea (which contain natural methylxanthines), are widely used to supplement, or replace, short-acting β-2 agonists (SABAs) for "rescue" treatment of acute asthma.[29,48,49] Adults also report the use of home remedies to augment asthma self-management, such as Hall's lozenge-infused tea (Mondelēz International Three Parkway North Deerfield, IL, USA), OTC chest rubs, and the ingestion of onion tonics, spicy foods (eg, horseradish), or cold drinks.[29] Importantly, a small number of individuals report oral ingestion of topical camphor products (eg, Vicks VapoRub [Proctor and Gamble, Cincinnati, Ohio, USA]).[29] Although few of these products have been scientifically evaluated, there are several studies of dietary supplements. These include studies of magnesium,[50] fish oil alone[51,52] or in combination with Vitamin C, and a standardized hops extract.[23] Asthma quality-of-life scores improved in those who received long-term magnesium supplementation[50] and the combined nutritional supplement (fish oil, Vitamin C, and hops).[23] However, there was no attention control group in the combination supplement study, making it impossible to attribute improvements to the supplement.[23] Other markers of asthma control, such as reduced bronchial hyperreactivity, pulmonary function, and inflammatory biomarkers improved with magnesium and fish oils.[50,51]

Potential Dangers of Natural Products for Pediatric and Adult Asthma

Several innocuous-appearing natural and OTC products have the potential for serious side effects, including death. For example, *Echinacea* (cone flower daisy) and chamomile are members of the Compositae or ragweed family. Worsening asthma may result if a ragweed-sensitive individual uses products derived from the daisy family, which includes honey made from the plants or pollens of Compositae.[53]

In addition, OTC natural ephedra (found in *ma huang*, a Traditional Chinese Medicine herb), can have a synergistic cardiovascular effect when used with albuterol.[54] Black licorice made from the glycyrrhiza root can prolong the half-life of cortisone, potentiating systemic steroid effects.[55] Further, the recommended dose of Hall's is 1 to 2 lozenges every 2 hours, which delivers a total dose of 6 to 20 mg of menthol; some adults used large quantities of lozenges (10) in a single serving of tea,[29] which may be harmful.[56]

Of greatest concern, however, were the reports of turpentine oil and Vicks VapoRub ingestion[29,44] and risky behaviors associated with natural product use. First, ingesting turpentine oil[57] and OTC topical chest rubs can be fatal in children and may pose some risk for adults.[58] Second, even when natural product use is not in and of itself harmful, its use may contribute to risky health behaviors. For example, herbal product use is associated with decreased inhaled corticosteroid adherence.[59] Further, substituting caffeinated products (tea and coffee) for SABAs translates to the use of less potent natural therapies for more rapid-acting and effective prescription therapies during acute asthma episodes.[37] This may lead to less effective reversal of bronchospasm and contribute to delays in seeking appropriate medical intervention, placing the individual at increased risk for near-fatal or fatal asthma.[41]

Mind-body Medicine

Mind-body medicine encompasses a wide variety of practices that seek to use the mind to enhance physical functioning and health and are generally considered safe in healthy people when practiced.[90] **Table 1** provides detailed information about many mind-body practices.

Mind-body Medicine for Pediatric Asthma

Breathing exercises (59%),[16] prayer (70%–80%),[33,60] and relaxation (85%) are the most popular mind-body approaches used by children with asthma.[33] Relaxation training may be taught as a stand-alone therapy[61,62] or paired with biofeedback[63,64] or guided imagery.[65–67] Although early studies suggested that relaxation might improve lung function,[62] these findings were not replicated in larger trials.[61] However, in several small feasibility studies without a control condition, biofeedback-induced relaxation was associated with improvement in lung function,[63,65,68] stress,[63] depression,[63] and anxiety,[65] whereas relaxation coupled with guided imagery improved lung function and anxiety.[66,67] Although one small RCT of biofeedback and relaxation demonstrated improved pulmonary function, anxiety, and attitudes toward asthma, there was no difference between groups in asthma medication use, number of asthma attacks, or self-concept.[64]

Hypnosis has also been examined in 2 pediatric asthma studies using a pre-post design. Reductions in symptoms[69] and severity scores without concomitant improvement in the number of asthma episodes or in pulmonary function tests were reported.[70] Further, a small RCT of an art therapy intervention (compared with a wait-list control) reported decreased anxiety and increased quality of life,[71] whereas music therapy (singing) was associated with maintenance or improvement of lung function compared with relaxation.[72]

Mind-body Medicine for Adult Asthma

Mind-body approaches are very popular among adults with asthma, including qi gong, tai chi,[11] prayer, humoral balance, and relaxation.[29,37] Intervention studies of relaxation have demonstrated improvement in well-being and pulmonary function, as well as reduced symptoms[73] without a reduction in cortisol after training.[74] Subjects enrolled in biofeedback[27] or guided (mental) imagery[75] interventions required less asthma medicine[27,75] and demonstrated improved lung function without concomitant improvement in the number of asthma flares[27] compared with a control group.

Other mind-body approaches studied included yoga, meditation, and music therapy. In a small controlled trial of yoga instruction that included postures (*yogasanas*), breathing exercises (*pranayamas*), and meditation, intervention subjects reported enhanced relaxation and less SABA use compared with control subjects, although objective measures of lung function remained unchanged.[76] Further, a randomized, controlled, double-masked clinical trial of Iyengar yoga failed to demonstrate any between-group differences in asthma quality of life, SABA use, spirometry, symptoms, or health care utilization for asthma.[26] In addition, small intervention studies of transcendental meditation,[77] music therapy, and progressive muscle relaxation[27] improved lung function, although the small increases in function were not considered to be of clinical significance.[27]

Two studies used multiple CAM interventions. In the first RCT, yoga, journaling, and nutritional manipulation (elimination diet coupled with supplements of fish oil, Vitamin C, and a standardized hops extract) were given to the intervention group with subsequent improvements in their asthma quality of life scores. These results should be viewed cautiously, however, because of the lack of a control group and the confounding of multiple interventions.[23] In the second study, patients with asthma received training on multiple mind-body approaches, including deep-breathing relaxation, a cognitive-behavioral intervention, and journaling. When compared with an attention control group, the intervention group experienced improved lung function.[78]

Single studies of Buteyko breathing and hypnotic susceptibility in adults have also been conducted. In an RCT of Buteyko, intervention subjects demonstrated improved asthma control with less medication use up to 6 months after training compared with the control condition.[79] Moreover, a correlational study identified that higher hypnotic susceptibility scores were associated with less airway hyperreactivity.[79]

Finally, several RCTs of acupuncture have been conducted in adults with asthma with mixed results. Treatment was associated with improved asthma quality of life[25] and reports of improved asthma[80] although acupuncture did not demonstrate improved lung function,[80,81] reduced need for medications,[25,81] or reduced symptoms.[81]

Potential Dangers of Mind-Body Medicine for Pediatric and Adult Asthma

NCCAM classifies most of the mind-body interventions as "safe"; however, there is small risk associated with some approaches. For example, progressive muscle relaxation has been associated with decreased airflow[82–84] and increased heart rate variability[82,83] in patients with asthma. In addition, there are case reports of untoward effects of mind-body therapies in the general population. For example, case reports describe complications related to yogic postures, including nerve or spinal damage,[85] worsened glaucoma,[86] and stroke.[87] There are also reports of yoga breathing causing pneumothorax.[88] Rare but serious complications may also result from acupuncture, including blood-borne illnesses, punctured organs, and vascular damage.[89] There are also reports of intensification of mania and distress after meditation[90] and hypnosis[91] in patients with mental illness.

Manipulative and Body-based Practices

Spinal manipulation and massage are the 2 primary manipulative and body-based approaches. As described further in **Table 1**, practitioners manipulate joints and massage soft tissue to reduce pain and stress and to facilitate relaxation.

Manipulative and Body-based Practices for Pediatric Asthma

There are very few studies of manipulative and body-based practices despite a high rate of use by children with asthma.[35] A small RCT demonstrated that massage therapy reduced anxiety and cortisol levels immediately after treatment and improved attitudes toward asthma and lung function over time compared with the control condition (progressive muscle relaxation). These findings were more pronounced in younger children compared with older children.[92] In a study by Bronfort and colleagues,[93] chiropractic spinal manipulative therapy improved asthma quality-of-life scores but failed to demonstrate any important changes in lung function or airway hyperreactivity compared with a sham chiropractic treatment. In an RCT of a spinal manipulation intervention, chiropractic care provided no additional benefit over usual medical care in children with mild to moderate asthma.[94]

Manipulative and Body-based Practices for Adult Asthma

Only one study of manipulative therapy (craniosacral treatment) for adults with asthma was identified in this review.[25] In this investigation, 89 subjects were randomized to 1 of 5 groups: acupuncture alone, craniosacral therapy alone, acupuncture and craniosacral therapy together, attention control, or usual care/wait list. Asthma quality-of-life scores improved in all 3 of the active intervention groups, although the combination of acupuncture and craniosacral treatment was not superior to either therapy alone. Medication use and pulmonary function were unchanged.[25]

Potential Dangers of Manipulative and Body-based Practices for Pediatric and Adult Asthma

When provided by a trained therapist, there are relatively few serious risks associated with massage or spinal manipulation for children or adults with asthma. Before massage therapy is initiated, a health care professional should provide medical clearance for individuals with concomitant conditions, such as pregnancy, propensity for bleeding (bleeding disorders, anticoagulant therapy), solid tumor cancers, blood clots, fractures, open wounds, skin infections, osteoporosis, or recent surgery.[95] Most serious side effects associated with spinal manipulation involve treatment of the cervical area and may include vertebrobasilar artery stroke and cauda equina syndrome.[96]

Whole Medical Systems for Asthma

Whole medical systems are complete systems of theory and practice that have evolved over time in different cultures and apart from Western medicine.[4] They include Traditional Chinese Medicine from China, Ayurveda from India, and homeopathy and naturopathy from Europe (see **Table 1**). Although these systems are widely used for asthma, no adult or pediatric studies were identified in this review.

Potential Dangers of Whole Medical Systems for Asthma

Mind-body medicine, manipulative approaches, and natural products are often essential components of whole medical systems approach to treating asthma. Therefore, the previous caution about their use is operative when patients seek such treatment; however, a particular point should be made about homeopathy. Because homeopathic treatments traditionally involve the ingestion of natural products, clinicians may be concerned about interactions or adverse side effects. Generally, plant material used in the preparation of homeopathic products is diluted to such infinitesimally small doses that not even one single active biologic molecule may remain in the "mother tincture," thus rendering the product harmless.[97] However, nasal zinc is an exception to this rule. Reports of permanent loss of smell forced the Food and Drug Administration to recall this homeopathic cold remedy, which was not neither dilute nor orally ingested.[98]

Energy Field Healing

As described in **Table 1**, magnets, Reiki, and therapeutic touch are the most commonly used energy-field healing practices. No adult or pediatric studies of energy healing were identified in this review.

Potential Dangers of Energy-Field Healing for Asthma

There is no known risk in the use of energy field healing practices such as Reiki or therapeutic touch.[99] Magnets are also safe when applied to the skin and are contraindicated only for individuals with medical devices affected by strong magnetic fields, such as pacemakers, implanted defibrillators, and insulin pumps.[100]

Movement Therapies

Pilates, Rolfing, and Alexander are common movement therapies (see detailed in **Table 1**). No adult or pediatric studies examining movement practices were identified in this review.

Potential Dangers of Movement Therapies for Asthma

Although only one scholarly article on the safety of movement therapies was located (a single case report of a spontaneous diaphragm rupture attributable to Pilates),[101] it is likely that some of the same concerns about massage may be applicable to Rolfing and that the Alexander technique might cause minor fatigue or muscle tenderness.

Traditional Healers

Mexican *Curandera*, Native American *shaman*, Puerto Rican *santeros,* and Voudoun *houngans* and *mambos* are among the many traditional healers that practice healing arts in North America (see **Table 1**). No adult or pediatric studies examining traditional healers were identified in this review.

Potential Dangers of Traditional Healers for Asthma

The use of natural products in traditional healing may cause drug-herb interactions, as previously described. In addition, some herbal preparations may be smoked as a treatment for asthma.[102] Alternatively, individuals may visit a smokehouse where poor indoor air quality has been identified as a health risk for individuals with respiratory disorders, including asthma.[103] Other potential dangers of traditional healing have not been reported.

CAM and Asthma Self-management Decisions and Behavior: Self-management Preferences, Adherence, and Patient-Provider Communication

This review uncovered important information, not only about the types and patterns of CAM use, but also about the influence of CAM on asthma self-management decisions and behaviors in children and adults with asthma. For instance, a large qualitative study found that mothers considered their child's daily asthma therapy to be optional despite it being prescribed for daily use, were strongly influenced by their social network to use CAM for their child's asthma, and were not demographically distinguishable from mothers who used conventional prescription treatment.[28] Most (77%) caregivers considered herbal therapies to be safe and did not believe that herbs interacted with medication; only 1% could correctly name a drug-herb interaction.[44]

Further, research demonstrated that adolescents were familiar with culturally relevant CAM[104] and believed CAM to be an effective part of their asthma armamentarium.[30,60] Conversely, 71% of children and their caregivers voiced concerns about the safety of prescription therapies.[43] However, self-reported adherence to daily asthma therapies did not change with the initiation of CAM.[105]

Despite the high rates of CAM use, only one-third of pediatricians asked about CAM.[106] Importantly, if asked, caregivers disclosed at relatively low rates ranging, from 36%[31] to 54%.[107] Caregivers were more comfortable disclosing yoga and dietary interventions than prayer or guided imagery.[33] As a result of this reluctance to divulge CAM use, partial disclosure was more common (62%).[35] However, 80% of caregivers reported that they wanted to tell their provider about their child's CAM use.[31]

Most adults (84%) preferred an integrated approach for asthma self-management that included CAM and prescription therapies.[37] Nurses and CAM practitioners were more likely to ask about CAM use than allopathic physicians,[108] although there are no disclosure rates available specific to adults with asthma. CAM use was associated with low rates of adherence to daily prescription medicines[37,59] and increased rates of hospitalization for life-threatening asthma.[49,59] These high rates of acute health care utilization were independent of disease severity, suggesting that the use of less potent CAM for the home management of acute asthma may unnecessarily delay professional treatment and contribute to higher hospitalization rates.[49] This is supported by qualitative studies in which patients reported that CAM was safe and effective for the initial treatment of severe attacks,[29] was safer than SABAs, worked quickly and synergistically with SABAs,[37] and allowed for the customized treatment the patients desired.[37,109]

SUMMARY

There is a growing body of evidence on the use of CAM by individuals with asthma, particularly in the domains of natural products, mind-body medicine, and manipulative and body-based practices. Natural products were the most common CAM used by both children and adults with asthma. Unfortunately, much of what is known about the effectiveness of these treatments is based primarily on prevalence surveys and a few methodologically weak intervention studies that reported mixed results. Of note, several natural OTC products have the potential for serious side effects, including death. Use of natural products was also associated with risky asthma self-management behaviors, such as decreased adherence to allopathic treatments.[59] Mind-body medicines were also frequently used for asthma with one-third of the reviewed literature focused uniquely on this CAM approach. There were also several trials of spinal manipulation and massage, examples of manipulative and body-based practices. Again, weak study designs, mixed results, and the possibility of serious side effects are concerning. Most importantly, CAM use was rarely discussed in the clinical encounter.

Many clinicians assume that patients turn to CAM only when they have received a cancer diagnosis or develop cancer treatment–related symptoms.[110,111] However, CAM is a popular treatment for asthma as well as a number of other chronic medical conditions, including diabetes,[5,6,111,112] hypertension,[5,6,113] and heart disease.[5,6,114] The desire to use CAM as a way of personalizing treatment has also been noted by other researchers.[115,116] Perhaps one of the most underappreciated risks of CAM is the failure of health care providers to inquire about CAM and patients' reluctance to disclose CAM use.[117]

There are several clinical implications of this review. First, it is important for clinicians and patients to discuss the risks associated with CAM use that include, but are not limited to, use of adulterated natural products, drug-herb interactions, and rare but serious events associated with innocuous-appearing therapies. Second, all CAM self-management strategies must be assessed for their timeliness and appropriateness, and negotiated through a shared decision-making model. For example, this review identified the risky behavior of substituting CAM for both "rescue" and daily asthma therapies. Perhaps a jointly developed plan that promotes the use of both CAM and prescription therapies at each of these events would be useful as a means of addressing patient preferences while also reducing the risk of an untoward event.

To be successful in this endeavor will require the provider to become better educated about CAM, to take the initiative in inquiring about CAM at each office visit, and to create a safe environment in which disclosure is facilitated. With this comes responsibility on the part of the health care professional to respond respectfully and professionally to disclosure. If the patient perceives that the provider is dismissive, derisive, or unsupportive, then a disruption to the therapeutic alliance can result.[118] Health care professionals need help to successfully meet these expectations. The construction and validation of research instruments that address the integral role of CAM in asthma self-management decisions is a critical first step in the systematic collection of data about patient perceptions and preferences for care.[119] Engaging in continuing education is also of paramount importance, as this training will facilitate a deeper appreciation for the reasons patients prefer CAM and will promote the acquisition of the enhanced communication skills needed to support integrative treatment as a cornerstone of patient-centered care.

In summary, this review provides clinicians with important new information: (1) CAM is widely used by both children and adults with asthma; (2) relatively little is known about the safety or effectiveness of CAM for asthma, owing to the paucity of well-designed studies; (3) patients use CAM to create a tailored asthma self-management plan; (4) CAM influences patients' prescription medication–taking behaviors, which, in turn, produces other health risks; and (5) patients and health care professionals do not talk about, or participate in, shared decision making concerning CAM use. Most importantly, this review identifies knowledge gaps that can be addressed by future research. Taken together, this new knowledge may help narrow the divide between what patients want, and what providers currently offer, for asthma self-management.

REFERENCES

1. Kleinman A, Eisenberg L, Good B. Culture, illness, and care: clinical lessons from anthropologic and cross-cultural research. Ann Intern Med 1978;88(2): 251–8.
2. Romanucci-Ross L. The hierarchy of resort in curative practices: the Admiralty Islands, Melanesia. In: Landy D, editor. Culture, disease, and healing: studies in medical anthropology. New York: Macmillan; 1977. p. 481–7.
3. World Health Organization. WHO traditional medicine strategy 2002–2005. 2002. Available at: http://elinks.library.upenn.edu/sfx_local?sid=Refworks%3AUniversity%20of%20Pennsylvani&charset=utf-8&__char_set=utf8&genre=article&aulast=World%20Health%20Organization&date=2002&volume=2012&issue=07%2F22&atitle=WHO%20traditional%20medicine%20strategy%202002%E2%80%932005.&au=World%20Health%20Organization%20&. Accessed July 22, 2012.

4. National Center for Complementary and Alternative Medicine. What is complementary and alternative medicine? 2012. Available at: http://elinks.library.upenn.edu/sfx_local?sid=Refworks%3AUniversity%20of%20Pennsylvani&charset=utf-8&__char_set=utf8&genre=article&aulast=National%20Center%20for%20Complementary%20and%20Alternative%20Medicine&date=2012&volume=2012&issue=07%2F22&atitle=What%20is%20complementary%20and%20alternative%20medicine%3F&au=National%20Center%20for%20Complementary%20and%20Alternative%20Medicine%20&. Accessed July 22, 2012.

5. Esmail N. Complementary and alternative medicine in Canada: trends in use and public attitudes 1997-2006. Public Policy Sources 2007;87:1–53.

6. Nahin RL, Barnes PM, Stussman BJ, et al. Costs of complementary and alternative medicine (CAM) and frequency of visits to CAM practitioners: United States, 2007. Natl Health Stat Report 2009;(18):1–14.

7. Barnes PM, Bloom B, Nahin RL. Complementary and alternative medicine use among adults and children: United States, 2007. Natl Health Stat Report 2008;(12):1–23.

8. Metcalfe A, Williams J, McChesney J, et al. Use of complementary and alternative medicine by those with a chronic disease and the general population—results of a national population based survey. BMC Complement Altern Med 2010;10:58.

9. Hannah L. Complementary and alternative medicine use among Mexican-Americans for general wellness and mental health. Master's thesis, Pacific University. 2010.

10. Barnes PM, Powell-Griner E, McFann K, et al. Complementary and alternative medicine use among adults: United States, 2002. Adv Data 2004;(343):1–19.

11. Torres-Llenza V, Bhogal S, Davis M, et al. Use of complementary and alternative medicine in children with asthma. Can Respir J 2010;17(4):183–7.

12. Polit D, Beck C. Nursing research: generating and assessing evidence for nursing practice. Philadelphia: Lippincott Williams & Wilkins; 2011.

13. Joubert A, Kidd-Taylor A, Christopher G, et al. Complementary and alternative medical practice: self-care preferred vs. practitioner-based care among patients with asthma. J Natl Med Assoc 2010;102(7):562–9.

14. Centers for Disease Control and Prevention. About the National Health Interview Survey. 2012. Available at: http://elinks.library.upenn.edu/sfx_local?sid=Refworks%3AUniversity%20of%20Pennsylvani&charset=utf-8&__char_set=utf8&genre=article&aulast=Centers%20for%20Disease%20Control%20and%20Prevention&date=2012&volume=2012&issue=27%2F07&atitle=About%20the%20National%20Health%20Interview%20Survey&au=Centers%20for%20Disease%20Control%20and%20Prevention%20&. Accessed July 27, 2012.

15. Knoeller GE, Mazurek JM, Moorman JE. Complementary and alternative medicine use among adults with work-related and non-work-related asthma. J Asthma 2012;49(1):107–13.

16. Shen J, Oraka E. Complementary and alternative medicine (CAM) use among children with current asthma. Prev Med 2012;54(1):27–31.

17. Marino LA, Shen J. Characteristics of complementary and alternative medicine use among adults with current asthma, 2006. J Asthma 2010;47(5):521–5.

18. Birdee GS, Wayne PM, Davis RB, et al. T'ai chi and qigong for health: patterns of use in the United States. J Altern Complement Med 2009;15(9):969–73.

19. Loera JA, Black SA, Markides KS, et al. The use of herbal medicine by older Mexican Americans. J Gerontol A Biol Sci Med Sci 2001;56(11):M714–8.

20. Bero L, Rennie D. The Cochrane Collaboration. Preparing, maintaining, and disseminating systematic reviews of the effects of health care. JAMA 1995; 274(24):1935–8.
21. Salim A, Mackinnon A, Griffiths K. Sensitivity analysis of intention-to-treat estimates when withdrawals are related to unobserved compliance status. Stat Med 2008;27(8):1164–79.
22. Lachin JL. Statistical considerations in the intent-to-treat principle. Control Clin Trials 2000;21(5):526.
23. Kligler B, Homel P, Blank AE, et al. Randomized trial of the effect of an integrative medicine approach to the management of asthma in adults on disease-related quality of life and pulmonary function. Altern Ther Health Med 2011; 17(1):10–5.
24. Covar R, Gleason M, MacOmber B, et al. Impact of a novel nutritional formula on asthma control and biomarkers of allergic airway inflammation in children. Clin Exp Allergy 2010;40(8):1163–74.
25. Mehl-Madrona L, Kligler B, Silverman S, et al. The impact of acupuncture and craniosacral therapy interventions on clinical outcomes in adults with asthma. Explore (NY) 2007;3(1):28–36.
26. Sabina AB, Williams AL, Wall HK, et al. Yoga intervention for adults with mild-to-moderate asthma: a pilot study. Ann Allergy Asthma Immunol 2005;94(5): 543–8.
27. Lehrer PM, Vaschillo E, Vaschillo B, et al. Biofeedback treatment for asthma. Chest 2004;126(2):352–61.
28. Freidin B, Timmermans S. Complementary and alternative medicine for children's asthma: satisfaction, care provider responsiveness, and networks of care. Qual Health Res 2008;18(1):43–55.
29. George M, Birck K, Hufford DJ, et al. Beliefs about asthma and complementary and alternative medicine in low-income inner-city African-American adults. J Gen Intern Med 2006;21(12):1317–24.
30. Reznik M, Ozuah PO, Franco K, et al. Use of complementary therapy by adolescents with asthma. Arch Pediatr Adolesc Med 2002;156(10):1042–4.
31. Ottolini MC, Hamburger EK, Loprieato JO, et al. Complementary and alternative medicine use among children in the Washington, DC area. Ambul Pediatr 2001; 1(2):122–5.
32. Cabana MD, Gollapudi A, Jarlsberg LG, et al. Parent perception of their child's asthma control and concurrent complementary and alternative medicine use. Pediatr Asthma Allergy Immunol 2008;21(4):167–72.
33. Cotton S, Luberto CM, Yi MS, et al. Complementary and alternative medicine behaviors and beliefs in urban adolescents with asthma. J Asthma 2011; 48(5):531–8.
34. Sidora-Arcoleo K, Yoos HL, McMullen A, et al. Complementary and alternative medicine use in children with asthma: prevalence and sociodemographic profile of users. J Asthma 2007;44(3):169–75.
35. Post-White J, Fitzgerald M, Hageness S, et al. Complementary and alternative medicine use in children with cancer and general and specialty pediatrics. J Pediatr Oncol Nurs 2009;26(1):7–15.
36. Ang JY, Ray-Mazumder S, Nachman SA, et al. Use of complementary and alternative medicine by parents of children with HIV infection and asthma and well children. South Med J 2005;98(9):869–75.
37. George M, Campbell J, Rand C. Self-management of acute asthma among low-income urban adults. J Asthma 2009;46(6):618–24.

38. Baldwin CM, Long K, Kroesen K, et al. A profile of military veterans in the southwestern United States who use complementary and alternative medicine: implications for integrated care. Arch Intern Med 2002;162(15):1697–704.

39. National Center for Complementary and Alternative Medicine. Time to talk about dietary supplements: 5 things consumers need to know. 2012. Available at: http://elinks.library.upenn.edu/sfx_local?sid=Refworks%3AUniversity%20of%20 Pennsylvani&charset=utf-8&__char_set=utf8&genre=article&aulast=National %20Center%20for%20Complementary%20and%20Alternative%20Medicine& date=2012&volume=2012&issue=07%2F25&atitle=Time%20To%20Talk%20 About%20Dietary%20Supplements%3A5%20Things%20Consumers%20Need %20To%20Know&au=National%20Center%20for%20Complementary%20and %20Alternative%20Medicine%20&. Accessed July 25, 2012.

40. National Center for Complementary and Alternative Medicine. Using dietary supplements wisely. 2012. Available at: http://elinks.library.upenn.edu/sfx_local? sid=Refworks%3AUniversity%20of%20Pennsylvani&charset=utf-8&__char_set= utf8&genre=article&aulast=National%20Center%20for%20Complementary%20 and%20Alternative%20Medicine&date=2012&volume=2012&issue=07%2F24 &atitle=Using%20Dietary%20Supplements%20Wisely&au=National%20Center %20for%20Complementary%20and%20Alternative%20Medicine%20&. Accessed July 24, 2012.

41. National Center for Complementary and Alternative Medicine. Safe use of complementary health products and practices. 2012. Available at: http://elinks.library. upenn.edu/sfx_local?sid=Refworks%3AUniversity%20of%20Pennsylvani& charset=utf-8&__char_set=utf8&genre=article&aulast=National%20Center% 20for%20Complementary%20and%20Alternative%20Medicine&date=2012& volume=2012&issue=07%2F25&atitle=Safe%20Use%20of%20Complementary %20Health%20Products%20and%20Practices&au=National%20Center%20for %20Complementary%20and%20Alternative%20Medicine%20&. Accessed July 25, 2012.

42. Milner JD, Stein DM, McCarter R, et al. Early infant multivitamin supplementation is associated with increased risk for food allergy and asthma. Pediatrics 2004; 114(1):27–32.

43. Handelman L, Rich M, Bridgemohan CF, et al. Understanding pediatric innercity asthma: an explanatory model approach. J Asthma 2004;41(2):167–77.

44. Lanski SL, Greenwald M, Perkins A, et al. Herbal therapy use in a pediatric emergency department population: expect the unexpected. Pediatrics 2003; 111(5 Pt 1):981–5.

45. Nahin RL, Fitzpatrick AL, Williamson JD, et al. Use of herbal medicine and other dietary supplements in community-dwelling older people: baseline data from the Ginkgo Evaluation of Memory study. J Am Geriatr Soc 2006;54(11):1725–35.

46. Hailemaskel B, Dutta A, Wutoh A. Adverse reactions and interactions among herbal users. Issues Interdiscipl Care 2001;3(4):297–300.

47. Zayas LE, Wisniewski AM, Cadzow RB, et al. Knowledge and use of ethnomedical treatments for asthma among Puerto Ricans in an urban community. Ann Fam Med 2011;9(1):50–6.

48. Blanc PD, Trupin L, Earnest G, et al. Alternative therapies among adults with a reported diagnosis of asthma or rhinosinusitis: data from a population-based survey. Chest 2001;120(5):1461–7.

49. Blanc PD, Kuschner WG, Katz PP, et al. Use of herbal products, coffee or black tea, and over-the-counter medications as self-treatments among adults with asthma. J Allergy Clin Immunol 1997;100(6 Pt 1):789–91.

50. Kazaks AG, Uriu-Adams JY, Albertson TE, et al. Effect of oral magnesium supplementation on measures of airway resistance and subjective assessment of asthma control and quality of life in men and women with mild to moderate asthma: a randomized placebo controlled trial. J Asthma 2010;47(1):83–92.

51. MacRedmond R, Singhera G, Attridge S, et al. Conjugated linoleic acid improves airway hyper-reactivity in overweight mild asthmatics. Clin Exp Allergy 2010;40(7):1071–8.

52. Mickleborough TD, Lindley MR, Ionescu AA, et al. Protective effect of fish oil supplementation on exercise-induced bronchoconstriction in asthma. Chest 2006;129(1):39–49.

53. National Center for Complementary and Alternative Medicine. Chamomile. 2011. Available at: http://elinks.library.upenn.edu/sfx_local?sid=Refworks%3AUniversity%20of%20Pennsylvani&charset=utf-8&__char_set=utf8&genre=article&aulast=National%20Center%20for%20Complementary%20and%20Alternative%20Medicine&date=2011&volume=2012&issue=07%2F25&atitle=Chamomile&au=National%20Center%20for%20Complementary%20and%20Alternative%20Medicine%20&. Accessed July 25, 2012.

54. Newall CA, Anderson LA, Phillipson JD. Herbal medicines: a guide for health-care professionals. London: The Pharmaceutical Press; 1996.

55. National Center for Complementary and Alternative Medicine. Licorice root. 2011. Available at: http://elinks.library.upenn.edu/sfx_local?sid=Refworks%3AUniversity%20of%20Pennsylvani&charset=utf-8&__char_set=utf8&genre=article&aulast=National%20Center%20for%20Complementary%20and%20Alternative%20Medicine&date=2011&volume=2012&issue=07%2F25&atitle=Licorice%20Root&au=National%20Center%20for%20Complementary%20and%20Alternative%20Medicine%20&. Accessed July 25, 2012.

56. Michael JB, Sztajnkrycer MD. Deadly pediatric poisons: nine common agents that kill at low doses. Emerg Med Clin North Am 2004;22(4):1019–50.

57. McKenzie LB, Ahir N, Stolz U, et al. Household cleaning product-related injuries treated in US emergency departments in 1990-2006. Pediatrics 2010;126(3):509–16.

58. Nair B. Final report on the safety assessment of Mentha piperita (peppermint) oil, Mentha piperita (peppermint) leaf extract, Mentha piperita (peppermint) leaf, and Mentha piperita (peppermint) leaf water. Int J Toxicol 2001;20(Suppl 3):61–73.

59. Roy A, Lurslurchachai L, Halm EA, et al. Use of herbal remedies and adherence to inhaled corticosteroids among inner-city asthmatic patients. Ann Allergy Asthma Immunol 2010;104(2):132–8.

60. Luberto CM, Yi MS, Tsevat J, et al. Complementary and alternative medicine use and psychosocial outcomes among urban adolescents with asthma. J Asthma 2012;49(4):409–15.

61. Alexander AB, Cropp GJ, Chai H. Effects of relaxation training on pulmonary mechanics in children with asthma. J Appl Behav Anal 1979;12(1):27–35.

62. Alexander AB, Miklich DR, Hershkoff H. The immediate effects of systematic relaxation training on peak expiratory flow rates in asthmatic children. Psychosom Med 1972;34(5):388–94.

63. Long KA, Ewing LJ, Cohen S, et al. Preliminary evidence for the feasibility of a stress management intervention for 7- to 12-year-olds with asthma. J Asthma 2011;48(2):162–70.

64. Kotses H, Harver A, Segreto J, et al. Long-term effects of biofeedback-induced facial relaxation on measures of asthma severity in children. Biofeedback Self Regul 1991;16(1):1–21.

65. Kapoor GV, Bray MA, Kehle TJ. School-based intervention: relaxation and guided imagery for students with asthma and anxiety disorder. Can J Sch Psychol 2010;25(4):311–27.
66. Dobson RL, Bray MA, Kehle TJ, et al. Relaxation and guided imagery as an intervention for children with asthma: a replication. Psychol Schools 2005;42(7):707–20.
67. Peck HL, Bray MA, Kehle TJ. Relaxation and guided imagery: a school-based intervention for children with asthma. Psychol Schools 2003;40(6):657–75.
68. Coen BL, Conran PB, McGrady A, et al. Effects of biofeedback-assisted relaxation on asthma severity and immune function. Pediatr Asthma Allergy Immunol 1996;10(2):71–8.
69. Anbar RD. Hypnosis in pediatrics: applications at a pediatric pulmonary center. BMC Pediatr 2002;2:11.
70. Kohen DP, Wynne E. Applying hypnosis in a preschool family asthma education program: uses of storytelling, imagery, and relaxation. Am J Clin Hypn 1997;39(3):169–81.
71. Beebe A, Gelfand EW, Bender B. A randomized trial to test the effectiveness of art therapy for children with asthma. J Allergy Clin Immunol 2010;126(2):263–6, 266.e1.
72. Wade LM. A comparison of the effects of vocal exercises/singing versus music-assisted relaxation on peak expiratory flow rates of children with asthma. Music Ther Perspect 2002;20(1):31–7.
73. Smyth JM, Soefer MH, Hurewitz A, et al. The effect of tape-recorded relaxation training on well-being, symptoms, and peak expiratory flow rate in adult asthmatics: a pilot study. Psychol Health 1999;14(3):487–501.
74. Smyth J, Litcher L, Hurewitz A, et al. Relaxation training and cortisol secretion in adult asthmatics. J Health Psychol 2001;6(2):217–27.
75. Epstein GN, Halper JP, Barrett EA, et al. A pilot study of mind-body changes in adults with asthma who practice mental imagery. Altern Ther Health Med 2004;10(4):66–71.
76. Vedanthan PK, Kesavalu LN, Murthy KC, et al. Clinical study of yoga techniques in university students with asthma: a controlled study. Allergy Asthma Proc 1998;19(1):3–9.
77. Wilson AF, Honsberger R, Chiu JT, et al. Transcendental meditation and asthma. Respiration 1975;32(1):74–80.
78. Hockemeyer J, Smyth J. Evaluating the feasibility and efficacy of a self-administered manual-based stress management intervention for individuals with asthma: results from a controlled study. Behav Med 2002;27(4):161–72.
79. Cowie RL, Conley DP, Underwood MF, et al. A randomized controlled trial of the Buteyko technique as an adjunct to conventional management of asthma. Respir Med 2008;102(5):726–32.
80. Wechsler ME, Kelley JM, Boyd IO, et al. Active albuterol or placebo, sham acupuncture, or no intervention in asthma. N Engl J Med 2011;365(2):119–26.
81. Tashkin DP, Kroening RJ, Bresler DE. A controlled trial of real and simulated acupuncture in the management of chronic asthma. J Allergy Clin Immunol 1985;76(6):855–64.
82. Aboussafy D, Campbell TS, Lavoie K, et al. Airflow and autonomic responses to stress and relaxation in asthma: the impact of stressor type. Int J Psychophysiol 2005;57(3):195–201.
83. Lehrer PM, Hochron SM, Mayne T, et al. Relationship between changes in EMG and respiratory sinus arrhythmia in a study of relaxation therapy for asthma. Appl Psychophysiol Biofeedback 1997;22(3):183–91.

84. Lehrer PM, Hochron SM, Mayne T, et al. Relaxation and music therapies for asthma among patients prestabilized on asthma medication. J Behav Med 1994;17(1):1–24.
85. Sinaki M. Yoga spinal flexion positions and vertebral compression fracture in osteopenia or osteoporosis of spine: case series. Pain Pract 2012. [Epub ahead of print].
86. Baskaran M, Raman K, Ramani KK, et al. Intraocular pressure changes and ocular biometry during Sirsasana (headstand posture) in yoga practitioners. Ophthalmology 2006;113(8):1327–32.
87. Duval EL, Van Coster R, Verstraeten K. Acute traumatic stroke: a case of bow hunter's stroke in a child. Eur J Emerg Med 1998;5(2):259–63.
88. Johnson DB, Tierney MJ, Sadighi PJ. Kapalabhati pranayama: breath of fire or cause of pneumothorax? A case report. Chest 2004;125(5):1951–2.
89. National Center for Complementary and Alternative Medicine. Acupuncture side effects, and risks. 2012. Available at: http://elinks.library.upenn.edu/sfx_local? sid=Refworks%3AUniversity%20of%20Pennsylvani&charset=utf-8&__char_set= utf8&genre=article&aulast=National%20Center%20for%20Complementary% 20and%20Alternative%20Medicine&date=2012&volume=2012&issue=07% 2F25&atitle=Acupuncture%20Side%20Effects%20and%20Risks&au=National %20Center%20for%20Complementary%20and%20Alternative%20Medicine% 20&. Accessed July 25, 2012.
90. National Center for Complementary and Alternative Medicine. Meditation: side effects and risks. 2012. Available at: http://elinks.library.upenn.edu/sfx_local? sid=Refworks%3AUniversity%20of%20Pennsylvani&charset=utf-8&__char_set= utf8&genre=article&aulast=National%20Center%20for%20Complementary% 20and%20Alternative%20Medicine&date=2012&volume=2012&issue=07%2F 25&atitle=Meditation%3A%20Side%20Effects%20and%20Risks&au=National %20Center%20for%20Complementary%20and%20Alternative%20Medicine% 20&. Accessed July 25, 2012.
91. Kluft RP. Issues in the detection of those suffering adverse effects in hypnosis training workshops. Am J Clin Hypn 2012;54(3):213–32.
92. Field T, Henteleff T, Hernandez-Reif M, et al. Children with asthma have improved pulmonary functions after massage therapy. J Pediatr 1998;132(5):854–8.
93. Bronfort G, Evans RL, Kubic P, et al. Chronic pediatric asthma and chiropractic spinal manipulation: a prospective clinical series and randomized clinical pilot study. J Manipulative Physiol Ther 2001;24(6):369–77.
94. Balon J, Aker PD, Crowther ER, et al. A comparison of active and simulated chiropractic manipulation as adjunctive treatment for childhood asthma. N Engl J Med 1998;339(15):1013–20.
95. National Center for Complementary and Alternative Medicine. Massage therapy: an introduction. 2012. Available at: http://elinks.library.upenn.edu/sfx_local? sid=Refworks%3AUniversity%20of%20Pennsylvani&charset=utf-8&__char_set= utf8&genre=article&aulast=National%20Center%20for%20Complementary%20 and%20Alternative%20Medicine&date=2012&volume=2012&issue=07%2F25 &atitle=Massage%20Therapy%3A%20An%20Introduction&au=National%20 Center%20for%20Complementary%20and%20Alternative%20Medicine%20&. Accessed July 25, 2012.
96. National Center for Complementary and Alternative Medicine. Chiropractic: an introduction. 2012. Available at: http://elinks.library.upenn.edu/sfx_local?sid= Refworks%3AUniversity%20of%20Pennsylvani&charset=utf-8&__char_set=utf8 &genre=article&aulast=National%20Center%20for%20Complementary%20and

%20Alternative%20Medicine&date=2012&volume=2012&issue=07%2F25& atitle=Chiropractic%3A%20An%20Introduction&au=National%20Center%20for %20Complementary%20and%20Alternative%20Medicine%20&. Accessed July 25, 2012.

97. National Center for Complementary and Alternative Medicine. Homeopathy: an introduction. 2012. Available at: http://elinks.library.upenn.edu/sfx_local? sid=Refworks%3AUniversity%20of%20Pennsylvani&charset=utf-8&__char_ set=utf8&genre=article&aulast=National%20Center%20for%20Complementary %20and%20Alternative%20Medicine&date=2012&volume=2012&issue=07% 2F25&atitle=Homeopathy%3A%20An%20Introduction&au=National%20Center %20for%20Complementary%20and%20Alternative%20Medicine%20&. Accessed July 25, 2012.

98. National Center for Complementary and Alternative Medicine. Time to talk about natural products for the flu and colds: what does the science say? 2012. Available at: http://elinks.library.upenn.edu/sfx_local?sid=Refworks%3AUniversity%20of% 20Pennsylvani&charset=utf-8&__char_set=utf8&genre=article&aulast=National %20Center%20for%20Complementary%20and%20Alternative%20Medicine&date= 2012&volume=2012&issue=07%2F25&atitle=Time%20To%20Talk%20About% 20Natural%20Products%20for%20the%20Flu%20and%20Colds%3AWhat% 20Does%20the%20Science%20Say%3F&au=National%20Center%20for% 20Complementary%20and%20Alternative%20Medicine%20&. Accessed July 25, 2012.

99. National Center for Complementary and Alternative Medicine. Reiki: an introduc-tion. 2012. Available at: http://elinks.library.upenn.edu/sfx_local?sid=Refworks% 3AUniversity%20of%20Pennsylvani&charset=utf-8&__char_set=utf8&genre= article&aulast=National%20Center%20for%20Complementary%20and%20Alter native%20Medicine&date=2012&volume=2012&issue=07%2F25&atitle=Reiki% 3A%20An%20Introduction&au=National%20Center%20for%20Complementary %20and%20Alternative%20Medicine%20&. Accessed July 25, 2012.

100. National Center for Complementary and Alternative Medicine. Magnets for pain. 2012. Available at: http://elinks.library.upenn.edu/sfx_local?sid=Refworks %3AUniversity%20of%20Pennsylvani&charset=utf-8&__char_set=utf8&genre= article&aulast=National%20Center%20for%20Complementary%20and%20Alter native%20Medicine&date=2012&volume=2012&issue=07%2F25&atitle=Mag nets%20for%20Pain&au=National%20Center%20for%20Complementary%20 and%20Alternative%20Medicine%20&. Accessed July 25, 2012.

101. Yang YM, Yang HB, Park JS, et al. Spontaneous diaphragmatic rupture compli-cated with perforation of the stomach during Pilates. Am J Emerg Med 2010; 28(2):259.e1–3.

102. University of Maryland Medical Center. Lobelia. 2010. Available at: http://elinks. library.upenn.edu/sfx_local?sid=Refworks%3AUniversity%20of%20Pennsylvani &charset=utf-8&__char_set=utf8&genre=article&aulast=University%20of%20 Maryland%20Medical%20Center&date=2010&volume=2012&issue=07%2F25 &atitle=Lobelia&au=University%20of%20Maryland%20Medical%20Center% 20&. Accessed July 25, 2012.

103. Flanagan ME, Zaferatos NC. Appropriate technologies in the traditional Native American smokehouse: public health considerations in tribal community devel-opment. Am Indian Cult Res J 2000;24(4):69–93.

104. Klein JD, Wilson KM, Sesselberg TS, et al. Adolescents' knowledge of and beliefs about herbs and dietary supplements: a qualitative study. J Adolesc Health 2005;37(5):409.

105. Philp JC, Maselli J, Pachter LM, et al. Complementary and alternative medicine use and adherence with pediatric asthma treatment. Pediatrics 2012;129(5):e1148–54.
106. Sawni A, Thomas R. Pediatricians' attitudes, experience and referral patterns regarding complementary/alternative medicine: a national survey. BMC Complement Altern Med 2007;7:18.
107. Sidora-Arcoleo K, Yoos HL, Kitzman H, et al. Don't ask, don't tell: parental nondisclosure of complementary and alternative medicine and over-the-counter medication use in children's asthma management. J Pediatr Health Care 2008;22(4):221–9.
108. Davis PA, Gold EB, Hackman RM, et al. The use of complementary/alternative medicine for the treatment of asthma in the United States. J Investig Allergol Clin Immunol 1998;8(2):73–7.
109. Mithani S, Monteleone C. Use of alternative therapies in patients with asthma in central New Jersey data from a pilot survey: data from a pilot survey. Journal of Asthma and Allergy Educators 2011;2(3):130–4.
110. Anderson JG, Taylor AG. Use of complementary therapies for cancer symptom management: results of the 2007 National Health Interview Survey. J Altern Complement Med 2012;18(3):235–41.
111. Vapiwala N, Mick R, Hampshire MK, et al. Patient initiation of complementary and alternative medical therapies (CAM) following cancer diagnosis. Cancer J 2006;12(6):467–74.
112. Nahas R, Moher M. Complementary and alternative medicine for the treatment of type 2 diabetes. Can Fam Physician 2009;55(6):591–6.
113. Nahas R. Complementary and alternative medicine approaches to blood pressure reduction: an evidence-based review. Can Fam Physician 2008;54(11):1529–33.
114. Greenfield S, Pattison H, Jolly K. Use of complementary and alternative medicine and self-tests by coronary heart disease patients. BMC Complement Altern Med 2008;8:47.
115. Edwards E. The role of complementary, alternative, and integrative medicine in personalized health care. Neuropsychopharmacology 2012;37(1):293–5.
116. Astin JA. Why patients use alternative medicine: results of a national study. JAMA 1998;279(19):1548–53.
117. Eisenberg DM, Kessler RC, Van Rompay MI, et al. Perceptions about complementary therapies relative to conventional therapies among adults who use both: results from a national survey. Ann Intern Med 2001;135(5):344–51.
118. Tasaki K, Maskarinec G, Shumay DM, et al. Communication between physicians and cancer patients about complementary and alternative medicine: exploring patients' perspectives. Psychooncology 2002;11(3):212–20.
119. Sidora-Arcoleo K, Feldman J, Serebrisky D, et al. Validation of the Asthma Illness Representation Scale (AIRS). J Asthma 2010;47(1):33–40.
120. Murphy AI, Lehrer PM, Karlin R, et al. Hypnotic susceptibility and its relationship to outcome in the behavioral treatment of asthma: some preliminary data. Psychol Rep 1989;65(2):691–8.

Asthma and Obesity: The Dose Effect

Amy B. Manion, PhD, RN, PNP[a,b,*]

KEYWORDS

- Asthma • Obesity • Dose effect

KEY POINTS

- Asthma is one of the most common chronic illnesses in the world, affecting an estimated 300 million people.
- Globally, the prevalence of asthma has continued to spread as economic improvements in developing countries create a population trend toward urbanization and adoption of a western lifestyle.
- Research supports an association between obesity and asthma.

As the populations of the world have evolved from a mainly rural, mainly agrarian society, to a more urban and industrial society, the challenges facing modern medicine have also evolved. What were once the mainstays of concern, infectious diseases, such as polio, tuberculosis, and typhoid, have now been replaced with an equally fatal, if not more insidious problem. As the new millennium begins, the high rate of mortality from infectious diseases has been replaced with chronic illnesses, such as heart disease, diabetes, and asthma.

ASTHMA

Asthma is one of the most common chronic illnesses in the world, affecting an estimated 300 million people.[1] Over the period 1980 through 1996, there was a dramatic increase in the prevalence of asthma among all ages, genders, and racial groups, especially in more urbanized nations such as the United States.[2] Currently, 24.6 million people living in the United States have been diagnosed with asthma.[3] Globally, the prevalence of asthma has continued to spread as economic improvements in developing countries create a population trend toward urbanization and adoption of a western lifestyle.[4,5] Based on this urbanization trend, it has been predicted that by

Funding Sources: Nil.
Conflict of Interest: Nil.
[a] Northwestern Children's Practice, Chicago, IL, USA; [b] College of Nursing, Rush University, 600 South Paulina Street, Chicago, IL 60612, USA
* Armour Academic Center, College of Nursing, Rush University, 600 South Paulina Street, 1080, Chicago, IL 60612.
E-mail address: Amy_manion@rush.edu

http://dx.doi.org/10.1016/j.cnur.2012.12.002
0029-6465/13/$ – see front matter © 2013 Elsevier Inc. All rights reserved.
nursing.theclinics.com

2025 an additional 100 million people will be diagnosed with asthma, increasing the global impact to 400 million.[1]

There is no cure for asthma. However, it can be controlled and managed with proper treatment. The general goals of asthma therapy consist of preventing chronic asthma symptoms and exacerbations, maintaining normal levels of activity, having normal or near-normal lung function, and having minimal side effects, while receiving optimal medication management.[6] Standard treatment of asthma consists of bronchodilators to relieve airway constriction, inhaled or oral corticosteroids to control inflammation, and avoidance of asthma triggers, such as smoke and other environmental irritants.[6]

Recently, combination therapy, consisting of an inhaled long-acting β_2-agonist along with an inhaled corticosteroid, has become the center of therapy for patients with moderate or severe persistent asthma.[7] In addition, leukotriene modifiers, which can prevent bronchoconstriction at a cellular level, are being used as add-on therapy.[7]

Despite the advances in therapeutic options, the economic burden of treating asthma in the United States has been expanding at an alarming rate because of the ever-increasing number of individuals diagnosed with the disease. In 1990, total costs due to asthma were estimated to be $6.2 billion.[8] By 1998, the cost of asthma had almost doubled to $11.3 billion, with direct costs accounting for $7.5 billion and indirect costs amounting to $3.8 billion.[9] Currently, the economic burden of asthma in the United States is staggering, with direct health care costs estimated at over $50 billion and indirect costs at $5.9 billion annually.[10]

Although asthma affects people of all ages, it disproportionately affects more children than adults, especially minority and poor children.[11,12] Currently, in the United States, over 10 million children and adolescents have been diagnosed with asthma, making it the leading chronic childhood illness.[13] Since 1999, children 5 to 17 years of age have demonstrated the highest prevalence rates with 109.3 per 1000 diagnosed with asthma, compared with 76.8 per 1000 in those over 18 years of age.[10] In 2009, the Centers for Disease Control and Prevention in the United States reported asthma prevalence ratios to be higher in children with approximately 1 in 12 for adults having asthma compared with 1 in 10 children.[14] The higher prevalence of asthma among children is not restricted to the United States; it is evident worldwide, especially in other industrial countries, such as the United Kingdom, where 1 in 7 children have been diagnosed with asthma compared with 1 in 25 adults.[15]

Furthermore, besides economic and age-related disparities, significant racial inequalities exist as well, especially in the more industrialized countries with the highest numbers of asthma prevalence. For example, in the United States, the asthma rate of prevalence is 43% higher for non-Hispanic blacks compared with non-Hispanic whites.[10] Even among children, these differences are evident. An analysis using results from the National Health Interview Survey 1997 to 2003 found that rate of asthma prevalence was consistently greater among non-Hispanic black children (15.7%) compared with non-Hispanic white children (11.5%) across all levels of income.[12] In addition, non-Hispanic black children are 3.6 times more likely to use the emergency department for asthma-related issues than non-Hispanic white children.[16] Multiple asthma-related emergency department visits are considered risk factors for fatal asthma, which is reflected in the rates of asthma mortality seen among minority groups, especially African Americans.[17] In 2006, non-Hispanic blacks had a rate of asthma mortality over 200% higher than non-Hispanic whites.[18] Furthermore, from 2003 to 2005, the Centers for Disease Control and Prevention reported that African American children had a rate of asthma mortality 7 times higher than non-Hispanic white children.[19] The World Health Organization has estimated the global rate of mortality from asthma to be 250,000 people annually.[20]

OBESITY

The high global prevalence of asthma and its continued drain on medical resources make it a major cause for concern. Nevertheless, another disturbing trend in health care use has revealed itself in the past decade as millions of American waistlines have grown to uncomfortable and unhealthy sizes. The prevalence of obesity in the United States is increasing at an alarming rate. Body mass index (BMI), defined as the weight in kilograms divided by the square of the height in meters, is commonly used to classify overweight and obesity among adults.[21] In adults, a BMI between 25 and 29.9 is defined as overweight, and a BMI of 30 or higher is considered obese. For children, overweight is defined as a BMI between the 85th and 94th percentile for age and gender, and obese is defined at a BMI at or above the 95th percentile for age and gender.[21]

According to data from the 2005 to 2006 National Health and Nutrition Examination Survey (NHANES), more than one-third of adults, or over 72 million people, are obese.[22] The incidence of obesity is increasing not only in the United States but also globally. Worldwide there are more than 1.5 billion overweight adults, with at least 500 million clinically obese adults.[23] The World Health Organization has predicted that by 2015, approximately 2.3 billion adults will be overweight and over 700 million will be obese.[24]

The worldwide increase in the prevalence of obesity is especially concerning because of the multitude of health problems associated with obesity. Obese and over-weight adults are at greater risk of cardiovascular disease, hypertension, stroke, type 2 diabetes, and certain forms of cancer, such as breast, pancreas, kidney, thyroid, and esophagus.[25] Approximately 85% of people with diabetes are type 2, and of these, 90% are overweight or obese.[23]

The true economic impact associated with the rise in obesity prevalence is difficult to determine due to the number of obesity-related conditions. The direct obesity-related medical costs in the United States have been estimated at $51.6 billion, whereas the indirect costs have been estimated at $47.6 billion.[26]

The increase in the prevalence of obesity in adults has been accompanied by a similar increase in the prevalence of obesity in children.[27] Furthermore, there is a strong cyclical relationship between adult and childhood obesity. For example, parental obesity more than doubles the risk of adult obesity in both obese and nonobese children.[28,29] If both parents are lean, a healthy child has a 14% chance of becoming overweight; however, if both parents are obese, the risk jumps to 80%.[30]

In the United States, the number of overweight children has doubled and the number of overweight adolescents has tripled over the last 2 decades.[31] The results from the 2003 to 2006 NHANES study showed an estimated 17% of children ages 6 to 11 years are overweight, which represents more than a 60% increase from the overweight estimates of 11% obtained from the 1988 to 1994 NHANES.[21]

The increasing prevalence of childhood overweight is not restricted to the United States alone. An estimated 22 million children under the age of 5 are considered over-weight worldwide.[24] Childhood overweight is becoming prevalent even in the developing world; for example, in Thailand, the prevalence of overweight in children 5 to 12 years of age increased from 12.2% to 15.6% in just 2 years.[23]

Similar to asthma, racial and ethnic disparities exist with obesity prevalence as well. In the United States, non-Hispanic blacks have a 51% higher rate of obesity, and

Hispanics have a 21% higher rate of obesity compared with non-Hispanic whites.[32] Similar to adults, NHANES data have shown the prevalence of obesity and overweight combined to be higher in non-Hispanic black children (35.4%) compared with non-Hispanic white children (28.2%).[33] The NHANES data found Mexican American boys ages 6 to 11 to have the highest combined obesity and overweight prevalence (43.9%).[33]

ASTHMA AND OBESITY

The increase in prevalence of both asthma and obesity has led to several studies examining the possible relationship between these 2 variables. Much of the research in this area has focused on the adult population. A study examining the trends in obesity among adults, using data from the NHANES I (1971–1975), II (1976–1980), and III (1988–1994), found that BMI increased universally among adults with asthma and those without; however, the prevalence of obesity rose more in the asthma group (21.3-32.8%) compared with the nonasthma group (14.6–22.8%).[34] A retrospective study of 143 individuals ages 18 to 88 found that the prevalence of obesity increased along with increasing asthma severity.[35]

The relationship between asthma and obesity demonstrated in studies conducted with adults has also been replicated in the pediatric population. A cross-sectional study using data from the Third National Health and Nutrition Examination Survey 1988 to 1994 showed that 2 of the highest risk groups for developing asthma were children over the age of 10 with a BMI greater than or equal to the 85th percentile (overweight and obese category) and children with a parental history of asthma who were 10 years or younger and of African American ethnicity.[36] A study conducted in the United Kingdom found that obesity among children 4 to 11 years of age was associated with asthma regardless of ethnicity, especially among girls.[37] Findings from the National Longitudinal Survey of Youth, which followed more than 4000 asthma-free children for 14 years, discovered a BMI at or greater than the 85th percentile at age 2 to 3 years was a risk factor for subsequent asthma development in boys.[38]

DOSE EFFECT

Research seems to support a relationship between obesity and asthma. Obesity has proven to be a risk factor for asthma in both adults and children.[39,40] There is a growing body of evidence to support a dose effect for asthma severity with obesity; however, a causal relationship has not been proven.

The evidence of a dose effect between obesity and asthma symptoms and severity is most strongly supported by the results from research conducted with patients who have experienced weight loss. In a study of 500 morbidly obese patients who underwent laparoscopic adjustable gastric banding surgery, greater than 80% of the patients who had asthma symptoms before surgery reported resolution or improvement in their symptoms.[41] A systematic review of studies examining asthma and weight loss found there was reversibility of at least 1 asthma outcome irrespective of whether weight loss was a result of surgical or medical intervention.[42] A meta-analysis of prospective studies involving obesity and asthma risk found asthma incidence increased by 50% in overweight and obese individuals regardless of gender, demonstrating a dose-dependent relationship between obesity and asthma.[43]

The dose effect relationship between obesity and asthma has also been researched in children. A study examining non-Hispanic black and Hispanic children age 2 to 18 years with asthma found the prevalence of overweight to be higher in children with moderate to severe asthma symptoms compared with the control group.[44] A more recent study found obese children with asthma used more asthma medications, wheezed more, and had a higher number of unscheduled emergency department visits than the nonobese children with asthma.[45] A large cross-sectional study of more than 400,000 adolescents found a significantly higher likelihood of asthma diagnosis occurring at higher BMI percentiles regardless of gender and race/ethnicity, indicating a positive dose response relationship between increasing BMI and asthma risk.[46]

Internationally, the dose effect relationship between obesity and asthma has also been documented. A large Norwegian study of more than 135,000 men and women found a 10% increase in asthma prevalence per unit of increase in BMI in men and a 7% increase in prevalence per unit increase in BMI in women.[47] A study in Taiwan of greater than 15,000 school-aged children found the prevalence of asthma increased as BMI elevated and high BMI coincided with low FEV_1/FCV scores on lung function testing, which is associated with lung impairment.[48] A similar result was found in a study conducted in Nova Scotia, Canada, that examined over 3000 students 10 to 11 years of age and found a linear association between BMI and asthma with a 6% increase in prevalence per unit increase of BMI.[49]

The exact mechanism creating the dose effect seen between obesity and asthma still needs further investigation. One theory proposed, which supports the less common view that asthma causes obesity, is that individuals with asthma restrict their levels of activity for fear of inducing an asthma exacerbation, which then leads to a more sedentary lifestyle and an increased risk of obesity.[37] Although many individuals with asthma might avoid vigorous physical activity and thus put on weight, this would seem, at best, an incomplete explanation for asthma causing obesity.[50]

The reverse association, that obesity causes asthma, and is the driving force behind the dose effect seen between these diseases has the most support. Proposed theories include mechanical, dietary, genetic, and hormonal.[46,51] One main theory that has generated the most discussion is the role pro-inflammatory cytokines such as leptin play in the process because adipose tissue is known as a primary source of these systemic immunomodulating agents and could be contributing to the chronic inflammation seen in asthma, creating more symptoms of the disease.[46,52] Cytokines are already believed to play a role in exercise-induced asthma, which could lead to proposals to add similar obesity-induced asthma nomenclature to the list of asthma categories.[53]

IMPLICATIONS

Whether the relationship between obesity and asthma is direct or indirect has yet to be determined. Nevertheless, the affects of obesity on asthma are evident and need to be incorporated into the management of the disease. Because prevention is the key to combating the steady rise in obesity, weight management should be addressed at each health care visit regardless of the individual's weight. For those individuals who are overweight or obese, nutritional counseling should be provided and a follow-up plan for weight loss should be developed. The positive effects of weight loss on asthma symptoms should be shared with patients to provide motivation and encouragement. Only by making weight management a priority in the treatment of asthma can the rising prevalence of both diseases be hindered and global health improved.

REFERENCES

1. Global Initiative for Asthma (GINA). The Global Strategy for Asthma Management and Prevention. 2011. Available at: http://www.Ginasthma.org/. Accessed June 15, 2012.

2. Akinbami LJ, Moorman JE, Garbe PL, et al. Status of childhood asthma in the United States, 1980–2007. Pediatrics 2009;123(Suppl 3):S131–45.
3. Centers for Disease Control and Prevention (CDC). Vital signs: asthma prevalence, disease characteristics, and self-management education: United States, 2001-2009. MMWR Morb Mortal Wkly Rep 2011;60(17):547–52 [0149-2195].
4. Bai J, Zhao J, Shen K, et al. Current trends of the prevalence of childhood asthma in three Chinese cities: a multicenter epidemiological survey. Biomed Environ Sci 2010;23:453–7.
5. Ait-Khaled N, Enarson DA, Bissell K, et al. Access to inhaled corticosteroids is key to improving quality of care for asthma in developing countries. Allergy 2007;62:230–6.
6. National Asthma Education and Prevention Program. Expert panel report 3: Guidelines for the diagnosis and management of asthma (No. NIH publication no. 07-4051). Bethesda (MD): National Heart Lung and Blood Institute; 2007.
7. Arellano FM, Arana A, Wentworth CE, et al. Prescription patterns for asthma medications in children and adolescents with health care insurance in the United States. Pediatr Allergy Immunol 2011;22:469–76.
8. Weiss KB, Sullivan SD. The health economics of asthma and rhinitis. Assessing the economic impact. J Allergy Clin Immunol 2001;107:3–8.
9. National Heart Lung and Blood Institute. Data fact sheet: asthma statistics. 1999. Available at: http://www.nhlbi.nih.gov/health/prof/lung/asthma/asthstat.pdf. Accessed March 3, 2006.
10. American Lung Association. Trends in morbidity and mortality. 2011. Available at: www.lung.org/finding-cures/our-research/trend-reports/asthma-trend-report.pdf. Accessed August 5, 2012.
11. Flores G, The Committee on Pediatric Research. Technical report- Racial and ethnic disparities in the health and health care of children. Pediatrics 2010; 125(4):e979–1021.
12. McDaniel M, Paxson C, Waldfogel J. Racial disparities in childhood asthma in the United States: Evidence from the National Health Interview Survey, 1997 to 2003. Pediatrics 2006;117(5):868–77.
13. Bloom B, Cohen RA, Freeman G. Summary health statistics for U.S. children: National health interview survey, 2010. Vital Health Stat 10 2010;(250):1–89.
14. CDC. 2011 Asthma in the U.S., Vital Signs. 2011. Available at: http://www.cdc.gov/VitalSigns/Asthma/. Accessed August 5, 2012.
15. Braman SS. The global burden of asthma. Chest 2006;130(1):4S–12S.
16. U.S. Department of Health and Human Services, Agency for Healthcare Research and Quality, National Healthcare Quality and Disparities Reports. 2011. Available at: www.ahrq.gov/qual/qrdr11/6_maternalchildhealth/T6_4_14_1_1.htm. Accessed June 19, 2012.
17. Carroll CL, Uygungil B, Zucker AR, et al. Identifying an at-risk population of children with recurrent near-fatal asthma exacerbations. J Asthma 2010;47:460–4.
18. CDC. Asthma prevalence, health care use and mortality: United States, 2003-2005. 2006. Available at: http://www.cdc.gov/nchs. Accessed August 15, 2009.
19. Akinbami LJ. The state of childhood asthma, United States, 1980-2005, Advance data from vital health statistics; no. 381. Hyattsville (MD): National Center for Health Statistics; 2006.
20. World Health Organization. Global surveillance, prevention and control of chronic respiratory diseases: a comprehensive approach. Geneva, Switzerland: World Health Organization; 2007.

21. CDC. Overweight and obesity. 2012. Available at: http://www.cdc.gov/obesity/adult/defining.html. Accessed June 19, 2012.
22. Ogden CL, Carroll MD, McDowell MA, et al. Obesity among adults in the United States- no change since 2003-2004. Hyattsville (MD): National Center for Health Statistics; 2007.
23. World Health Organization. Obesity and overweight. 2011. Available at: http://www.who.int/mediacentre/factsheets/fs311/en/index.html. Accessed July 6, 2012.
24. World Health Organization. WHO: global database on body mass index. 2012. Available at: http://www.who.int/bmi/index.jsp. Accessed July 6, 2012.
25. Kopelman P. Health risks associated with overweight and obesity. Obes Rev 2007;8(Suppl 1):13–7.
26. Li Z, Bowerman S, Heber D. Health ramifications of the obesity epidemic. Surg Clin North Am 2005;85(4):681–701.
27. Maffeis C, Tato L. Long-term effects of childhood obesity on morbidity and morality. Horm Res 2001;55(Suppl 1):42–5.
28. Krebs NF, Jacobson MS, American Academy of Pediatrics Committee on Nutrition. Prevention of pediatric overweight and obesity. Pediatrics 2003;112(2):424–30.
29. Whitaker RC, Wright JA, Pepe MS, et al. Predicting obesity in young adulthood from childhood and parental obesity. N Engl J Med 1997;337(13):869–73.
30. Hagarty MA, Schmidt C, Bernaix L, et al. Adolescent obesity: Current trends in identification and management. J Am Acad Nurse Pract 2004;16(11):481–9.
31. U.S. Preventative Services Task Force. Screening and interventions for overweight in children and adolescents: recommendation statement. Pediatrics 2005;116(1):205–9.
32. CDC. Differences in prevalence of obesity among black, white, and hispanic adults–United States, 2006-2008. MMWR Morb Mortal Wkly Rep 2009;58(27):740–4.
33. Wang Y, Beydoun MA. The obesity epidemic in the United States—Gender, age socioeconomic, racial/ethnic, and geographic characteristics: A systemic review and meta-regression analysis. Epidemiol Rev 2007;29:6–28.
34. Ford ES, Mannino DM. Time trends in obesity among adults with asthma in the United States: findings from three national surveys. J Asthma 2005;42(2):91–5.
35. Akerman MJ, Calacanis CM, Madsen MK. Relationship between asthma severity and obesity. J Asthma 2004;41(5):521–6.
36. Rodriguez MA, Winkleby MA, Ahn D, et al. Identification of population subgroups of children and adolescents with high asthma prevalence: findings from the Third National Health and Nutrition Examination Survey. Arch Pediatr Adolesc Med 2002;156(3):269–75.
37. Figueroa-Munoz JI, Chinn S, Rona RJ. Association between obesity and asthma in 4-11 year old children in the U.K. Thorax 2001;56:133–7.
38. Mannino DM, Mott J, Ferdinands JM, et al. Boys with high body masses have an increased risk of developing asthma: findings from the National Longitudinal Survey of Youth (NLSY). Int J Obes 2006;30(1):6–13.
39. Guerra S, Sherrill DL, Bobadilla A, et al. The relation of body mass index to asthma, chronic bronchitis, and emphysema. Chest 2002;122:1256–63.
40. Hjellvik V, Tverdal A, Furu K. Body mass index as predictor for asthma: a cohort study of 118, 723 males and females. Eur Respir J 2010;35(6):1235–42.
41. Spivak H, Hewitt MF, Onn A, et al. Weight loss and improvement of obesity-related illness in 500 U.S. patients following laparoscopic adjustable gastric banding procedure. Am J Surg 2005;189(1):27–32.

42. Eneli IU, Skybo T, Camargo CA Jr. Weight loss and asthma: a systematic review. Thorax 2008;63:671–6.
43. Beuther DA, Sutherland ER. Overweight, obesity, and incident of asthma. Am J Respir Crit Care Med 2007;175:661–6.
44. Luder E, Melnik TA, DiMaio M. Association of being overweight with greater asthma symptoms in inner city black and Hispanic children. J Pediatr 1998; 132(4):699–703.
45. Belamarich PF, Luder E, Kattan M, et al. Do obese inner-city children with asthma have more symptoms than nonobese children with asthma? Pediatrics 2000; 106(6):1436–41.
46. Davis A, Lipsett M, Milet M, et al. An association between asthma and BMI in adolescents: results from the California Healthy Kids survey. J Asthma 2007;44: 873–9.
47. Nystad W, Meyer HE, Nafstad P, et al. Body mass index in relation to adult asthma among 135,000 Norwegian men and women. Am J Epidemiol 2004;160:969–76.
48. Chiu YT, Chen WY, Wang TN, et al. Extreme BMI predicts higher asthma prevalence and is associated with lung function impairment in school-aged children. Pediatr Pulmonol 2009;44:472–9.
49. Sithole F, Douwes J, Burstyn I, et al. Body mass index and childhood asthma: a linear association? J Asthma 2008;45:473–7.
50. Shaneen SO. Obesity and asthma: cause for concern? Clin Exp Allergy 1999; 29(3):291–3.
51. Chin S. Obesity and asthma: evidence for and against a causal relation. J Asthma 2003;40(1):1–16.
52. Silva P, Mello M, Cheik N, et al. The role of pro-inflammatory and anti-inflammatory adipokines on exercise-induced bronchospasm in obese adolescents undergoing treatment. Respir Care 2012;57(4):572–82.
53. Hallstrand TS, Moody MW, Aitken ML, et al. Airway immunopathology of asthma with exercise-induced bronchoconstriction. J Allergy Clin Immunol 2005;116(3): 586–93.

Asthma in the Workplace

Laura Lemmenes, MS/MBA, APN, DNP

KEYWORDS

- Asthma • Workplace • Occupational asthma • Work-related asthma

KEY POINTS

- Several factors, both occupational and nonoccupational, will influence the development of occupational asthma (OA).
- Although much more study focused on OA needs to be completed, it can be stated with some surety that identification of IgE-mediated sensitization and bronchial hyperresponsiveness occurs with OA.
- Extreme short-term chemical exposures versus a cumulative effect of chemical exposures will need continued evaluation to determine tolerable levels that do not cause harm. Population-based surveys continue in occupations, such as animal facilities, farming, bakeries, seafood processing plants, carpet and latex glove manufacturing, plastic and varnish production, and the pharmaceutical and hospital industries.
- Health care providers often seek guidance from NIOSH, which sponsors ongoing research and training related to workplace exposures.

Occupational asthma (OA), also known more broadly as work-related asthma (WRA), refers to asthma that occurs as a result of workplace inhalation exposures. This disease was first described centuries ago but the exact definition has been more difficult to obtain.[1,2] WRA is now the most common occupational lung disease in developing countries. Workplace exposures to physical or chemical agents may result in an exacerbation of a known preexisting asthma diagnosis or may be asthma induced by inhalation within the workplace. WRA has been implicated in up to 15% of all cases of asthma in adults within industrialized nations.[3–5] Asthma occurring from workplace exposures is often unrecognized and underestimated. Because of the nature of the disease and the disabling effects that can occur, it is imperative to identify the offending agents quickly and remove or protect the worker from further exposure.[6,7]

Work-related respiratory illnesses in particular have decreased in industrialized nations. This includes illnesses such as coal miner disease or black lung disease, asbestosis, and silicosis, all known as pneumoconiosis. Improved understanding of these conditions has led to use of proper precautions, as mandated by organizations, such as National Institute for Occupational Safety and Health (NIOSH). It should be noted, however, that WRA prevalence and incidence has been on the increase, often

Advocate Health Care, Advocate Medical Group, Occupational Health Orland Park Center, 9550 West 167th Street, Orland Park, IL 60467, USA
E-mail address: laura.lemmenes@advocatehealth.com

Nurs Clin N Am 48 (2013) 159–164
http://dx.doi.org/10.1016/j.cnur.2012.12.004
0029-6465/13/$ – see front matter © 2013 Elsevier Inc. All rights reserved.

nursing.theclinics.com

thought to be the result of new chemicals and processes used in production.[8,9] Epidemiologic studies found to be most useful in identifying this diagnosis include the population-based study that includes both single and multiple exposures to the agents. This design appears to have the most advantages, least limitations, and the ability to obtain the most information. There is no loss of subjects due to those leaving the work place, no bias related to mandatory physician reporting and eliminates the variety of OA definitions.[5]

Determining asthma symptoms and relationship between the symptoms and work is the first step. Evaluation of the worker should include the following:

- Changes in the work processes exposing the worker to offending agents or continuous exposure to agents causing a latent period of sensitization.
- Acute exposure to irritant agents within the past 24 hours.
- Asthma symptoms improve on weekends or periods away from work.
- Allergic rhinitis symptoms more prevalent while at work.

CATEGORIES OF WORK RELATED ASTHMA

There are 2 major divisions of WRA as noted in **Fig. 1**: OA and work-exacerbated asthma (WEA). WEA refers to the individuals who have a diagnosis of asthma and are found to have increased symptoms at work. There are 2 major classifications of OA. These include sensitizer-induced asthma and irritant-induced asthma. Sensitizer-induced asthma occurs after a latency period following exposure to a causal agent. This is also described as immunologic occupational asthma. Immunologic occupational asthma is described as accounting for 90% of the cases of OA. Irritant-induced asthma or nonimmunologic asthma refers to individuals without a preexisting diagnosis of asthma (also known as reactive airway dysfunction) who have a sudden reaction to the respiratory system by an offending irritant.[5,10–12] It is important to note that once the diagnosis of asthma has been made, along with standard treatments for asthma control, the provider should also consider providing work restrictions, avoiding triggers, and instituting environmental controls, such as a respirator or other personal protective equipment (PPE). With irritant-induced asthma, it may be important to avoid use of powdered inhaled agents, as found in various corticosteroid and bronchodilator preparations, as these may produce increased irritation.[3]

SENSITIZER INDUCED ASTHMA

There are more than 350 known sensitizers, both natural and synthetic chemicals, that have been identified within the workplace and have the potential to cause immunologic occupational asthma. These agents fall into 2 categories: low molecular weight

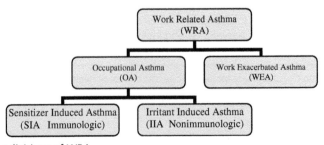

Fig. 1. Major divisions of WRA.

and high molecular weight agents. High molecular weight agents are proteins of animal or vegetable origin. Low molecular weight agents include organic and inorganic compounds. The most important determinant of this type of asthma is the amount or accumulation of the exposure. Immunoglobulin E (IgE) antibody responses have occurred following high exposure levels of know sensitizers, mainly from the high molecular weight agents. Unfortunately, identifying IgE-mediated responses to high molecular weight agents in the workplace is not always indicative of the development of immunologic occupational asthma. Studies of an exposure to red cedar between 2 cohorts identified IgE antibodies but did not have a cause-and-effect relationship with asthma symptoms.[10] Other agents commonly identified include flour; cereals; animal and insect allergens from fur/hair, saliva, urine, or dander; detergent, pharmaceutical, and baking enzymes, as well as natural latex rubber used in the health care field.[5,13]

Low molecular weight irritants are incomplete antigens. They combine with a protein to form a sensitizing neoantigen, unlike high molecular weight irritants. Low molecular weight chemicals are found in the manufacture of acid anhydrides and isocyanates found in polyurethane, plastics, epoxy, cleaning agents; platinum salts found in jewelry; acetic acid in soldering flux; plicatic acid in Western red cedar used by carpenters, wood carvers, and furniture makers; and persulfate salts used by hairdressers. Some workers are exposed to multiple sensitizers, such as health care workers. They are exposed to latex, cleaning agents, synthetic plaster cast material, orthopedic adhesives, sterilization fluids, and metals in dental alloys.

Sensitizer-induced asthma develops after a latency period in which the worker has been exposed to varied levels of a sensitizer. Following this period of sensitization, there are overt signs of asthma response. Pathophysiology behind the IgE mechanism is suspected to give rise to a cascade of events resulting in inflammatory cell activation and the release of inflammatory mediators. The presence of eosinophils, lymphocytes, and mast cells with thickening of the basement membrane has been identified, and is similar to what is found in the irritant-induced asthma.[5]

The primary route of exposure remains inhalation through the respiratory tract to the lungs; however, some agents have been identified as occurring through skin exposure and causing inflammatory lung changes, as well as IgE-mediated responses. Humans dermally exposed to methylene diphenyl diiocyanate (MDD) have been shown to develop the IgE-mediated responses with asthmatic reactions. MDD is used in the production of rigid polyurethane, which is a good thermal insulator and is used in refrigerators and freezers. This chemical is also used in high-strength glue preparations.

IRRITANT INDUCED ASTHMA

Irritant-induced asthma or nonimmunologic asthma was previously not considered occupational asthma. Irritant-induced asthma now is identified as occurring from a single exposure or multiple exposures to an irritant substance at a high concentration. Reactive airways dysfunction syndrome (RADS) is now considered a subset of this and is related to a single high concentration exposure. RADS which occurs following a high concentration exposure of an irritant agent, often from an occupational accident, and has been identified as occupationally related under the condition that there is a direct correlation between the inhalation exposure and the onset of asthma symptoms. This can occur with exposure to high concentrations of chlorine gas, anhydrous ammonia, or conditions that occurred similar to those following the collapse of the World Trade Center Towers in New York in 2001.[6,13] The World Trade Center cough was first described following exposure to inorganic highly alkaline dust, flammable materials, and other materials from the falling towers. Whether or not the cough was present, one-quarter of the firefighters experienced airway hyperrespon-siveness/bronchospasm. Those workers with initial airway hyperresponsiveness/bronchospasm continued to demonstrate RADS as demonstrated in a longitudinal study.[5]

The pathophysiology behind irritant-induced asthma following high levels of expo-sure is not completely understood. It is thought that there is an initial bronchial epithelial injury that then impairs the epithelial function, leading to epithelial cell release of inflammatory mediators. This release is followed by activation of nonadrenergic, noncholinergic pathways, neurotransmitter release, and resulting inflammation. This cascade is thought to trigger macrophage activity and mast cell degranulation, occur-ring with proinflammatory chemotactic and toxic mediators as a result of irritant expo-sures. Following the inflammatory response, remodeling of the airways occurs with subepithelial thickening and alteration of the mucous glands. Low irritant concentra-tion exposure is thought to cause bronchospasm.[6]

Host susceptibility appears to be a critical factor in the diagnosis of OA. This was observed when not all of the individuals exposed to the various agents developed OA. Therefore, additional risk factors associated with OA have been recognized. Atopy in the workers exposed to high molecular weight agents has been identified as a predis-posing factor, but this is a weak predictor of sensitization and further diagnosis of OA. Cigarette smoking has also been found to have an association with development of OA in those exposed to specific agents. Platinum salt exposure in cigarette smokers has a positive correlation with sensitization and development of OA. Most of these cases are mild in contrast to the severity of disease associated with cigarette smoking alone.[5]

Gender is shown to play a role in the distribution of occupational respiratory diseases most often attributable to the specific occupations and agents each sex is exposed to. For example, women are often exposed to cleaning agents with men more often exposed to agents found in welding-related occupations. Worker genetics is currently being studied as a predisposition to OA. This area of study will have many ethical, legal, and social ramifications.[5]

WORK RELATED ASTHMA

WRA should be considered in individuals with a diagnosis of asthma that is worsening or an individual who develops a new diagnosis of asthma as an adult. A complete work history looking for potentially causative agents or contributing factors is necessary. Onset, timing, and severity of symptoms related to work should be evaluated. This will include the type of job, exertion at work, extremes of temperature, ventilation, any current use of protective equipment, and respiratory diseases in coworkers. The magnitude and timing of exposures should be identified and documented. If a suspect chemical is identified, a literature search should follow and the Material Data Safety Sheet (MSDS) sheet should be made available to the employee. This will allow the employee and provider the ability to determine more about the potential irritant. MSDS sheets can then be used to perform a complete literature search to find additional information, as the MSDS may omit important data.[12] Identification of asthma that is worsened by work exposures may be more difficult to detect. Careful evaluation of putative chemical triggers may pinpoint the work relatedness. Continued exposure is often associated with worsening symptoms, diminished lung function, and poor overall outcomes. This identification is important for eliminating or controlling the exposure. Also, complicating the diagnosis of OA can be the transient nature of some employees. Distinguishing OA for workers has ramifications for medical/legal purposes mainly related to worker's compensation.[6,14]

EVALUATION OF WORKPLACE ASTHMA

Objective testing in the form of pulmonary function testing with Spirometry may provide some objective information as to the work-relatedness of the symptoms. Using the spirometer to evaluate for the values associated with WRA airflow obstruction while off work for 1 to 2 weeks and comparing with values obtained after working and coming in contact with the offending chemicals can in certain situations make a strong case for or against WRA. For individuals with the possibility of sensitizer-induced asthma, immunologic skin testing can be performed. This will identify specific work allergens that the individual is sensitive to.[12]

Differential diagnosis should be considered also. This may include vocal cord dysfunction, upper respiratory tract irritation, and psychogenic factors.

As noted earlier, eliminating or controlling the exposure in the workplace is of utmost importance once WRA has been diagnosed. In some situations, limiting the exposure to the offending agent may result in resolution of symptoms. This can be accomplished through engineering controls, such as improved ventilation and personal protective equipment (PPE), including the use of a dust mask or respirator. Engineering controls including the monitoring of airborne exposure levels should be considered. For those with topical exposures resulting in OA symptoms, wearing long sleeves or barrier sleeves may prevent further symptoms. Along with these changes, optimizing medical management may minimize or eliminate symptoms.

If symptoms cannot be minimized or eliminated, it is important to identify who will need to be removed from the specific work area if exacerbation of symptoms continues. The provider and the employee must carefully evaluate the potential benefit versus the potential risks, both long and short term, that may occur in the workplace setting. Employers may not discriminate against workers with WRA and are expected by the Equal Employment Opportunity Commission (EEOC) to provide good faith "reasonable" accommodations. If reasonable accommodations cannot be made, then the employee may not be able to work in that position. If an employee is identified in a post-offer employment examination to have chemical triggers that will be present in the job setting, it is in the best interest of the potential employee to practice primary prevention and possibly exclude that individual from the job, especially if PPE is not available.[14] Post-offer employment is often based on successfully passing the preemployment examination. Secondary prevention includes increased awareness of workers exposed to potential sensitizers through the use of respirator questionnaires and periodic pulmonary function testing with Spirometry.[6]

Individual worker prognosis is dependent on timely diagnosis, and removal or cessation of exposure to the offending agent. This becomes the responsibility not only of the employer but of the exposed worker. Identification by the employee, with truthful responses on respirator questionnaires will assist in the proper diagnosis and management of WRA.

Most workers exposed to antigens and irritants will not develop OA. Other factors both occupational and nonoccupational will influence the development of OA. Although much more study focused on OA needs to be completed, it can be stated with some surety that identification of IgE-mediated sensitization and bronchial hyper-responsiveness occurs with OA.[8] Also, extreme short-term chemical exposures versus a cumulative effect of chemical exposures will need continued evaluation to determine tolerable levels that do not cause harm. Population-based surveys continue in occupations such as animal facilities, farming, bakeries, seafood-processing plants, carpet and latex glove manufacturing, plastic and varnish production, and the pharmaceutical and hospital industries.[13] Health care providers often seek guidance from NIOSH, which sponsors ongoing research and training related to workplace exposures.

REFERENCES

1. Quirce S, Bernstein J. Old and new causes of occupational asthma. Immunol Allergy Clin North Am 2011;31(4):677–98.
2. Søyseth V, Johnsen HL, Henneberger PK, et al. The incidence of work-related asthma-like symptoms and dust exposure in Norwegian smelters. Am J Respir Crit Care Med 2012;185(12):1280–5.
3. Cowl C. Occupational asthma. Chest 2011;139(3):674–81.
4. Centers for Disease Control and Prevention (CDC). Work-related asthma—38 states and District of Columbia, 2006–2009. MMWR Morb Mortal Wkly Rep 2012;61(20):375–8.
5. Mapp CE, Boschetto P, Maestrelli P, et al. Occupational asthma. Am J Respir Crit Care Med 2005;172(3):280–305.
6. Dykewicz MS. Occupational asthma: current concepts in pathogenesis, diagnosis, and management. J Allergy Clin Immunol 2009;123(3):519–28 [quiz: 529–30].
7. Le Moual N, Kauffmann F, Eisen EA, et al. The healthy worker effect in asthma: work may cause asthma, but asthma may also influence work. Am J Respir Crit Care Med 2008;177(1):4–10.
8. Gautrin D, Newman-Taylor AJ, Nordman H, et al. Controversies in epidemiology of occupational asthma. Eur Respir J 2003;22(3):551–9.
9. Kanwal R. Severe occupational lung disease from exposure to flavoring chemicals. Am Fam Physician 2009;79(2):87.
10. Maestrelli P, Boschetto P, Fabbri LM, et al. Mechanisms of occupational asthma. J Allergy Clin Immunol 2009;123(3):531–42 [quiz: 543–4].
11. Malo JL, Chan-Yeung M. Agents causing occupational asthma. J Allergy Clin Immunol 2009;123(3):545–50.
12. Tarlo SM, Balmes J, Balkissoon R, et al. Diagnosis and management of work-related asthma: American College Of Chest Physicians Consensus Statement [review]. Chest 2008;134(Suppl 3):1S–41S [Erratum appears in Chest 2008;134(4):892].
13. Chan-Yeung M, Malo JL. Occupational asthma: definitions, epidemiology, causes, and risk factors. 2012. Available at: http://www.uptpdate.com/contents/occupational-asthma-definitions-epidemiology-causes-ad-risk-factors. Accessed August 16, 2012.
14. Henneberger PK, Mirabelli MC, Kogevinas M, et al. The occupational contribution to severe exacerbation of asthma. Eur Respir J 2010;36(4):743–50.

Management of Pediatric Asthma at Home and in School

Linda Sue Van Roeyen, MS, CSN, CCRP, FNP-BC

KEYWORDS

- Asthma • Pediatrics • Chronic inflammatory disorder • Shortness of breath

KEY POINTS

- The incidence of pediatric asthma in the United States creates a huge financial burden to the economy as well as a negative impact on child health.
- The management of asthma in the home and school is positively impacted through improved education for children, their families, and all those who care for them.
- Identification and elimination of asthma triggers are helpful in reducing asthma exacerbations.
- The incidence of asthma is higher in African American and underserved populations.
- Improved management of pediatric asthma leads to improved school performance, improved mental health, and general well-being.

Asthma is a chronic inflammatory disorder of the airways affecting adults and children of all ages. Asthma symptoms include shortness of breath, wheezing, coughing, and chest tightness. The single greatest risk factor for developing asthma in infants and children is the genetic predisposition for allergic diseases that includes atopic dermatitis and allergies. The Tucson Birth Cohort[1] identified the existence of eczema as a major risk factor in predicting the likelihood of persistent disease. Viral illnesses and previous infection with respiratory syncytial virus are also known to be risk factors. The asthma predictive index was developed from the Tucson Birth Cohort and provides major and minor criteria for the asthma predictive index. Major risk factors include parental asthma and physician-diagnosed atopic dermatitis. Minor risk factors include physician-diagnosed allergic rhinitis, wheezing unrelated to colds, and blood eosinophilia (>4%).[1]

According to the summary data from the 2010 National Health Institute Survey,[2] currently 7 million children or 9.6% of the pediatric population (less than 18 years of age) in the United States suffer from asthma. Asthma incidence is higher in the northeast and midwest United States geographically and, among women and children, African Americans, and persons with income below the level of poverty.[2,3]

Ann & Robert H. Lurie Children's Hospital of Chicago, Pulmonary Habilitation Program, Box 246, 225 East Chicago Avenue, Chicago, IL 60611, USA
E-mail address: Lvanroeyen@luriechildrens.org

Nurs Clin N Am 48 (2013) 165–175
http://dx.doi.org/10.1016/j.cnur.2012.12.006
0029-6465/13/$ – see front matter © 2013 Elsevier Inc. All rights reserved.

nursing.theclinics.com

Medical costs, hospitalizations, and emergency room visits for asthma are estimated at $50.1 billion per year.[3] Some costs include $3.8 billion in loss of productivity resulting from missed days of school or work, and $2.1 billion from lost productivity due to premature death.[4] In 2008 persons with acute asthma exacerbations missed an average of 4.5 days of school or work per year.[5] According to Healthy People 2020, 132.7 emergency room visits for asthma per 10,000 children less than the age of 5 occurred in 2005 to 2007 and 41.4 hospitalizations for asthma per 10,000 children less than the age of 5 occurred in 2007. The goals of Healthy People 2020 include promotion of respiratory health through better prevention, detection, treatment, and education efforts. The Healthy People 2020 goals related to asthma include the following: reduce asthma-related deaths, reduce asthma-related hospitalizations, reduce emergency department visits for asthma, reduce the proportion of persons who miss work or school days, and increase the proportion of persons with current asthma who receive appropriate asthma care according to National Asthma Education and Prevention Program Expert Panel Review 3 guidelines.[6] Established in 2007, the Expert Panel Review 3 guidelines focus on 4 areas of asthma care aimed at improving the quality of care and health outcomes. These guidelines include assessment and monitoring, patient education, control of factors contributing to asthma severity, and medical treatment. The guidelines report that inhaled corticosteroids are the most consistently effective long-term control medications for asthma management.[7] Pediatric health management of asthma requires coordination between a child's health care providers, school, and home. Children with asthma receive care in multiple settings from multiple persons: parents, caregivers, coaches, and teachers, who have variable knowledge and skills in asthma recognition and management. Children spend 7 hours or more per day in school. Therefore, it is extremely important to provide tools for the caregivers and teachers to assist in asthma management. The quality of life in children with asthma causes a negative impact on how they see themselves and how they interact with their peers and environment. Educational programs aimed at home and school management provide an excellent opportunity to decrease the rates of morbidity and mortality related to pediatric asthma.

ASTHMA IN THE HOME

The environmental triggers in the home significantly impact the quality of life of a child with asthma. Eliminating asthma triggers can be a key factor in decreasing exacerbations. Motivated and educated parents can learn to identify and eliminate or modify exposure to triggers and decrease the incidence of asthma flare-ups in their children. Commoon triggers include the following: exposure to cold air, viral illnesses, exercise, food allergies, pet dander, house dust mites, cockroaches, tobacco smoke, air pollution, perfumes, cleaning fluids, lead-based paints, mold, and pollen. Bronchoconstriction and increased airway inflammation are a result of the increased immunoglobulin E (in response to allergen exposure), which activates the release of mast cells. Repeated exposure to allergens can lead to worsening symptoms.[7] Parents should be taught to eliminate, to the extent possible, the triggers causing exacerbations. Elimination of triggers may include more frequent cleaning in the home with nonirritating chemicals. Pets may be confined to common family areas, and removed from the bedrooms, to provide decreased exposure for at least 8 to 10 hours per day. Pillowcases and mattress covers made to decrease allergens also assist in decreasing the effect of dust mites. Identification of food allergies for children greater than 2 years of age can be obtained through skin testing by a pediatric allergist and may assist in an avoidance of food allergy triggers. Identification and subsequent avoidance of food allergies are helpful in decreasing asthma symptoms. Promoting a clean, smoke-free environment, with the least amount of irritants, is helpful for the child with asthma.

CASE MANAGEMENT

Case management is another approach in promoting guideline care for asthma. In 2011 a study investigated the implementation of nurse case management and housing interventions to reduce allergen exposures. This study, known as the Milwaukee Randomized Controlled Trial,[8] included 121 children with asthma. The control group (n = 64) received a visual assessment, asthma education, bed/pillow dust mite encasings, and treatment of lead-based paint hazards. In addition, the interventions group (n = 57) received the following: nurse case management, which consisted of a tailored, individual asthma action plan; minor home repairs; home cleaning using special vacuuming and wet washing; and integrated pest management. The study concluded that nurse case management and home environmental interventions, while increasing collaboration between health and housing professionals, were effective in decreasing exposures to allergens such as settled dust; however, it was difficult to change home behavior related to food storage and disposal of food debris.[8] The use of case management in managing children with asthma and their home environmental condition has proven to be helpful. The use of emergency visits for pediatric patients was evaluated in 2010.[9] In this study, children with asthma received a home environmental assessment as recommended by a pediatric allergist as part of a comprehensive case management program. Findings showed that having a home environmental assessment and case manager may decrease medical care use for children suffering from allergic rhinitis and asthma.[9]

HOME INTERVENTIONS—ENVIRONMENT AND EDUCATION

Barriers to obtaining proper asthma management in families of low income must be first identified to provide relief. Barriers to asthma management include the following: lack of allergy assessment and treatment, pessimistic parental beliefs regarding their ability to impact the disease, parental mental health problems, lack of health knowledge and inappropriate expectations for care, lack of access to a consistent health care professional, and competing household priorities.[10] Effective interventions include educating families and children to empower them to manage their disease.

Environmental conditions related to asthma morbidity were reviewed in a Michigan study evaluating the use of a program called Healthy Homes University (HHU) that was implemented for low-income families. The program assessed homes for asthma triggers and provided products and services to reduce exposures to triggers. Education was provided to families including identification of triggers and specific behaviors to reduce exposures. The study included 243 caregivers at baseline and at 6 months. HHU implemented several of the objectives from Healthy People 2010 into their educational program. HHU reduced levels of indoor allergen through home visits by providing asthma trigger reduction products to households and educated caregivers regarding how to decrease indoor allergens. HHU improved substandard housing though correction of physical housing problems including water leaks, electrical deficiencies, pest infestation, inoperable heating equipment, and peeling lead-based paint. HHU reduced the population's exposure to pesticides through education of households about integrated pest management techniques and provided them with traps, baits, food containers, and trash cans. Asthma symptoms were significantly reduced and acute care visits for asthma decreased by more than 47%.[11] A Canadian study enrolled 398 children and families into 2 groups to investigate the use of interactive education in a small group and the effect on asthma control by children and their families. The intervention group showed much improved asthma control, significantly fewer visits to the emergency room, and improvements in their quality-of-life scores. Education in a small group proved to be very effective in improving asthma management and decreasing acute episodes.[12]

The effectiveness of a low-cost approach to improve control of asthma symptoms in an urban population through lay educators was reviewed in 2008. The study concluded that low cost in-home education and environmental remediation improved outcomes for children with asthma. Lay educators were effective in delivering asthma-specific education, which resulted in improved asthma control.[13]

A pilot study of a home-based family intervention for low-income children with asthma was conducted in 2012. Low-income African American children have disproportionately higher rates of asthma morbidity and mortality. This study examined 43 families from an urban hospital and asthma camp, enrolling children aged 8 to 13 who had poorly controlled asthma. These children were randomized to a 4- to 6-session Home-Based Family Intervention or a single session of Enhanced Treatment As Usual. The Home-Based Family Intervention looked at family-selected goals targeting asthma management and stressors. Families were given an asthma action plan and dust mite covers. Children performed spirometry and demonstrated metered-dose inhaler/spacer technique at each home visit. Results suggest that home-based intervention addressing medical and psychosocial needs may prevent hospitalizations for children with poorly controlled asthma and parents/caregivers under stress.[14] Another important consideration when examining barriers is cultural sensitivity. The development of a program geared at the Latino children in urban areas provided improved asthma management. A 2008 study examined the experience of being an Asthma Amigo, a community-based educator who delivered asthma education to a Hispanic community using a train-the-trainer educational model. Focus groups evaluated participant experiences and program strengths and weaknesses. Findings suggested this program helped in highlighting asthma triggers and prevention in this population.[15]

A program called CALMA (an acronym of the Spanish for "Take Control, Empower Yourself, and Achieve Management of Asthma") was trialed in Puerto Rico. It provided a culturally adapted family-based intervention for decreasing asthma morbidity in poor Puerto Rican children aged 5 to 12 with persistent asthma. Puerto Rican children have the highest rates of asthma of any ethnic group and are more likely to die from asthma when compared with other children. When evaluating the educational intervention, Puerto Rican families had less asthma exacerbations and used fewer services after the CALMA program was implemented. Conclusions demonstrated that providing a culturally adapted program for families and tailoring the needs of low-income Puerto Rican families decreased asthma morbidity in the children.[16]

Parents frequently do not receive adequate information to help their children manage their asthma symptoms. Average clinic appointments last from 20 to 45 minutes with little time for in-depth discussion of asthma teaching. Different types of asthma education programs for parents were examined. A Web-based program, "My Child's Asthma," provides interactive tools for parents to become more engaged in learning about their child's disease. A 2011 study looked at 283 parents with children who had asthma. Surveys examined demographic and clinical characteristics, outcome expectations, and self-efficacy beliefs regarding asthma control for their child and attitudes about computers and the Internet.

Results suggest it would be beneficial to find ways to increase engagement in a Web-based intervention for parents who are not yet engaging in recommended behaviors and/or those who report less positive outcome and efficacy expectations around asthma.[17]

PSYCHOSOCIAL/QUALITY OF LIFE

Asthma in the presence of other chronic medical illnesses is a concern for increased morbidity with asthma. Caregivers may have a positive impact on the health and well-being of children with medical and psychiatric comorbidities.[18] In a 2009 study examining the effect of routines on asthma management and rates of morbidity, outcomes for children with asthma and their parents were investigated. One hundred fifty children were enrolled and given quality-of-life scores comparing those with more versus those with less household routines, concluding that those with established routines may result in improved asthma morbidity outcomes.[19] In this systematic review, 16 studies measured quality-of-life issues in children or adolescents with asthma. The studies demonstrated an overall decrease of 0.8 symptom days in a 2-week period, or 21.0 fewer symptom days per year.[20] Allowing the child to participate in the clinic visit with parental coaching may be very helpful in solidifying the child's knowledge of their own asthma management plan. The goal for school-aged children is to change the dyadic interactions between the parent and provider into a triadic interaction, to include the child and thereby to improve their asthma management.[21] Shared decision-making in health care between the school-aged child and parents or medical professionals may also increase self-confidence and improve self-management skills.

ASTHMA IN THE SCHOOL
Absenteeism

Children with uncontrolled asthma are unable to perform at their best, and therefore, are at a disadvantage scholastically.[22] Identifying children with asthma and participating in their plan of care provide opportunities and challenges for the school system. School nurses play an important role in the care of asthmatic children in the creation and implementation of the care plan. However, many schools do not have school nurses on the premises and depend on office personnel to assist children with asthma management.[22,23] The School Health Policies and Programs Study of the Centers for Disease Control and Prevention assesses school health policies and programs at the state, district, school, and classroom levels. Their survey found that only 36% of schools have a full-time registered nurse or licensed practical nurse.[24] In some schools the school nurse is expected to maintain the attendance data and record keeping. Absence, extended absence, and repeated tardiness may occur because of asthma status. In a 2011 study by Mizan and coworkers, the mean days of absence in 86 students with asthma was 2.73 days compared with 1.89 days for 828 children without asthma. There was no difference in the number of days tardy. Students with asthma were more likely to be absent on Monday, Tuesday, and Friday than students without asthma.[22] Increased absenteeism may lead to decreased self-esteem and poor school performance. Subsequently, it may restrict future education and career opportunities.[4] The relationship between school absence, academic performance, and asthma status was examined in a predominantly African American urban school district. Children with absenteeism due to asthma symptoms did not test as well on standardized testing as those without asthma-related absenteeism.[23] Children with asthma are also more likely to be treated for mental health problems and demonstrate more negative social outcomes as well as decreased overall health and well-being.[25] Children with asthma who have parents with chronic disease show worsening health management and more absenteeism. It is important to understand how parents' health conditions influence children's health care and limit the child's participation in school and other activities.[26]

School-based Health Centers/Access to Care

The development of school-based health clinics (SBHC) may be the answer to providing improved asthma and general health care for the underserved. The National Association of School-based Health Centers has issued a policy statement identifying the implementation of SBHC to provide a medical home to provide primary care to this population.[27] The current health legislation provides for expansion of SBHC to provide primary care for children. The Patient Protection and Affordable Care Act (P.L.111–148), signed into law by President Obama in March 2012, provides language authorizing a federal SBHC grant program for operations, and an emergency appropriation that would provide $200 million for SBHC construction and equipment needs over 4 years. Provision of a funded federal program for SBHC will allow improved access to care for children and adolescents. Patient Protection and Affordable Care Act (Section 4101[a]) of the Affordable Care Act allows for SBHCs to access $200 million in competitive federal funds over the next 4 years. The grants are limited to facilities expenditures, such as the acquisition or improvement of land, construction costs, equipment, and similar expenditures. HR 1214 was passed in May 2011, by the House of Representatives, and provides for defunding of grants for SBHCs. Legislators are monitoring the pending of this law passing the senate and being signed by the President before it will go into effect.[27] SBHC currently provide onsite care by physicians or nurse practitioners in more than 1500 public schools in the United States. Revised National Institutes of Health, National Heart, Lung, and Blood Institute guidelines for the diagnosis and management of asthma provide evidence of the effectiveness of school-based programs to improve self-managed treatment of asthma among children.[24] The cost savings of implementing SBHC nationwide were reviewed. The costs considered not only the amount it would take to staff the SBHC, but also the cost savings of premature deaths, savings from absenteeism due to lost productivity for parents in the workplace, savings from decreased hospital costs, hospital costs at discharge for asthmatic school-aged children, medical costs for outpatient or physician office visits, decrease in emergency room use, actual cost of nursing salaries, actual emergency room use in acute asthma, and future earnings including fringe benefits and financial losses due to parent's need to stay home from work and provide care for the child at home. Medical savings alone did not offset the cost of implementing this program for asthma prevention. The reduction in asthma severity was estimated to save $260 million per year in emergency room and inpatient hospital costs.[28]

The Law

Liability for schools regarding asthma management and self-administration of medication may be of concern in many school districts. Because asthma attacks can occur without warning and require immediate emergency medication, children require access to their short-acting bronchodilators immediately. A delay in obtaining the medication may result in a required hospitalization or death. If a child needs to go to the nurse's office or principal to obtain the inhaler, this increases the risk for poor outcomes. Children with asthma should carry their rescue inhaler for facilitation of prompt administration. Several laws protect the right of children to carry emergency medications on their persons. These laws include the Individuals with Disabilities Education Act, Section 504 of the Rehabilitation Act of 1973, and Title III of the Americans with Disabilities Act.

The Individuals with Disabilities Education Act partly funds states to develop special education programs for children with disabilities. Children with asthma can be considered under the "other health impairment" section of the law, which would mandate that the school needs to meet the unique needs of the child and allow them to carry their inhaler. In the 504 plan of the Rehabilitation Act of 1973, discrimination is not allowed based on a disability. This plan defines individuals with a disability as someone with a "physical or mental impairment which substantially limits one or more major life activity and has a record of such impairment or is regarded as having such impairment."[29] By federal law, schools must make reasonable accommodations for children to carry their inhalers or have immediate access.

Last, Title III of the Americans with Disabilities Act provides public accommodations for people with disabilities in the private sector and for state and local entities that do not receive federal funding. Therefore, private schools would fall under this law and provide for nondiscrimination of students with disabilities in private schools.

Unfortunately, many school districts may be unaware of the laws and how they apply to children in school. It is necessary for the school nurse, and in some cases the parent, to serve as the child advocate to enlighten school districts of their legal responsibilities with regard to asthma management. School districts may need to adjust their policies to become updated with current laws allowing children to carry asthma medications. Some states have provided that, to comply with the federal law, state legislation identifies certain conditions must be met. For example, they require written authorization for parent or guardian for self-administration of asthma medication, a written statement from a licensed provider containing the student name, purpose, appropriate usage, dosage, time or times and under what circumstances the medication may be administered, and that the student has demonstrated the ability and understanding to self-administer the medication by passing an assessment by the school nurse who evaluates technique and level of understanding of the medication. In addition, the school district required parent acknowledgment in writing that they understand they will hold harmless the school, employees, agents, and school board from any injury resulting from self-administration of the medication.[29] In 2010 all 50 states agreed to allow the portability of asthma/allergy medication for children.[30] This agreement has allowed children to carry their rescue inhalers to class, lunch, and gym. Having a rescue inhaler available during known periods of possible asthma exacerbations improves access to care and decreases the incidence of asthma emergencies.

The school environment provides an excellent opportunity to screen for asthma in an effort to identify undiagnosed children and to deliver educational programs for children with asthma. Educating the teachers is extremely effective in decreasing the number of acute asthmatic episodes in children. Teachers may be the first to recognize early onset of a child who experiences respiratory distress/wheezing and requires short-acting bronchodilators per metered-dose inhaler with a spacer or even nebulized treatments in an effort to prevent an emergency room visit. In providing school-based asthma education, it is important to include the school personnel as well as children and families. The importance of providing an asthma-friendly school environment to provide improved asthma control was reviewed in 2008. Families need to be aware of school policies and procedures to navigate the school system better and to facilitate administration of medications while at school. Cicutto[31] suggests 8 goals to improve asthma management in school. The goals include the following:

1. Identify and track all students with asthma;
2. Assure immediate access to medications as prescribed;
3. Use an individualized asthma action plan for all students with asthma;
4. Encourage full participation in school-related activities, including physical activity;
5. Use standard emergency protocols for worsening asthma;
6. Educate all school personnel and students;
7. Identify and reduce common asthma triggers; and
8. Ensure communication and collaboration among school personnel, families, and health professionals/medical home, including discussion of asthma-related policies in school.

Immediate access to inhalers and an individualized asthma action plan give children the best possible opportunity to prevent acute exacerbations and to control them if they begin.[31]

Educational Programs in Schools

Multiple programs for schools have been studied to determine the best strategy for education in the school system. "Happy Air" is a school-based program for children and their families in primary grades with asthma. Children (n = 2765) and families were enrolled in the program that included diagnosis, clinical follow-up, education, self-management, and quality-of-life control aims to decrease the socioeconomic burden of asthma disease. Asthma management was significantly improved after the use of the program. An assessment to evaluate the need for educational programs was performed in 2010.[32] Findings showed that teachers' knowledge about asthma and asthma management is limited, especially among those whose students did not have active asthma. A more proactive approach to asthma management was recommended.[33] In the pilot testing, "Okay with Asthma," available at www.okay-with-asthma.org,[34] school-aged children aged 8 to 11 participated in an online asthma intervention program. This online asthma intervention program was originally developed for school nurses to use in health offices. The program was free and accessible to any school with Internet access. The self-guided program used a 20-minute animated story about a school-aged girl with asthma. It was used to convey asthma management strategies, including psychosocial strategies to adjust to asthma and the role of school personnel and peers in helping a child adjust to asthma. The efficacy of this program is not known, but could be replicated in larger samples over a longer period of time to learn the retention of asthma knowledge.[35] A review by Jones and colleagues looked at "How Asthma Friendly is Your School?" The questionnaire assessed 8 school health program components: health education, health services, physical education and activity, mental health and social services, nutrition services, healthy and safe school environment, faculty and staff health promotion, and family and community involvement. Administering this questionnaire highlighted the needs of the school system to provide additional programs for not only children and families but also all school ancillary personnel. Through the identification of deficiencies, improved educational programs can be implemented.[36]

Consulting Physician Role in Schools

Schools that have a consulting physician available provide improved asthma management and decrease absenteeism. It is hypothesized that parents have more confidence in the decisions of the school nurse when a consulting physician is in place.

In addition, school nurses have more self-confidence when they have the option of consulting with a physician regarding asthma treatment options. The 2009 study reviewing the implementation of a consulting physician in schools for children with asthma showed a decrease in absenteeism. The number of missed school days for students decreased from 8.9 to 7.5 after implementing the role of the consulting physician. The decreased absenteeism translates to increased reimbursement by school districts. More information is needed to examine the economic impact of implementing the consulting physician in school districts.[37]

SUMMARY

The incidence of pediatric asthma in the United States creates a huge financial burden to the economy as well as a negative impact on child health. The management of asthma in the home and school is positively impacted through improved education for children, their families, and all those who care for them. Identification and elimination of asthma triggers are helpful in reducing asthma exacerbations. The incidence of asthma is higher in African American and underserved populations. The implementation of effective asthma education improves the economic consequences for society and improves the health and future of children. Improved management of pediatric asthma leads to improved school performance and improved mental health and general well-being. The knowledge of the school nurse regarding federal and state laws is very helpful in providing improved asthma management for children. The use of an asthma action plan decreases the number of acute asthma exacerbations in children. It is the responsibility of the school nurse to educate school staff and ancillary personnel to assist in promoting child health and decreasing the health issues related to pediatric asthma.

REFERENCES

1. Stewart LJ. Pediatric asthma. Prim Care Clin Office Pract 2008;35:25–40.
2. CDC. National health Interview Survey (NHIS) data: 2008 lifetime and current asthma. Atlanta (GA): US Department of Health and Human Services, CDC; 2010. Available at: http://www.cdc.gov/asthma/nhis/08data.htm. Accessed August 6, 2012.
3. Barnett SB, Nurmagambetov TA. Costs of asthma in the United States: 2002-2008. J Allergy Clin Immunol 2011;127:145–52.
4. Crawford D. Understanding childhood asthma and the development of the respiratory tract. Nurs Child Young People 2011;23(7):25–34.
5. Centers for Disease Control and Prevention (CDC). Vital signs: asthma prevalence, disease characteristics, and self-management education. United States, 2001-2009. MMWR Morb Mortal Wkly Rep 2011;60:547–52.
6. Available at: http://www.healthypeople.gov/2020/topicsobjectives2020/objectiveslist.aspx?topicld=36. Accessed August 6, 2012.
7. National Institutes of Health, National Heart, Lung and Blood Institute (NHLBI). Guidelines for the diagnosis and management of asthma (EPR-3). Bethesda (MD): US Department of Health and Human Services, National institutes of health, National heart, Lung, and Blood Institute; 2007. Available at: http://www.nhlbi.nih.gov/guidelines/astha/asthgdln.pdf. Accessed August 8, 2012.
8. Breysse J, Wendt J, Dixon S, et al. Nurse case management and housing interventions reduce allergen exposures: the Milwaukee randomized controlled trial. Public Health Rep 2011;126(Suppl 1):89–99.

9. Barnes CS. Reduced clinic, emergency room, and hospital utilization after home environmental assessment and case management. Allergy Asthma Proc 2010; 31(4):317–23.
10. Davis D, Gordon M, Burns B. Educational interventions for childhood asthma: a review and integrative model for preschoolers from low-income families. Pediatr Nurs 2011;37(1):31–8.
11. Largo T, Borgialli M, Wisinski C, et al. Healthy Homes University: a home based environmental intervention and education program for families with pediatric asthma in Michigan. Public Health Rep 2011;126(Suppl 1):14–26.
12. Watson WT, Gillespie C, Thomas N, et al. Small group interactive education and the effect on asthma control by children and their families. CMAJ 2009;181(5): 257–63.
13. Bryant-Stephens T, Li Y. Outcomes of a home-based environmental remediation for urban children with asthma. J Natl Med Assoc 2008;100(3):306–16.
14. Celano MP. Home based family intervention for low income children with asthma a randomized controlled pilot study. J Fam Psychol 2012;26(2):171–8.
15. Lobar S. The experience of being an Asthma Amigo in a program to decrease asthma episodes in Hispanic children. J Pediatr Nurs 2008;23(5):364–71.
16. Canino G, Vila D, Normand S, et al. Reducing asthma health disparities in poor Puerto Rican children: the effectiveness of a culturally tailored family intervention. J Allergy Clin Immunol 2008;121(3):665–70.
17. Meischke H. Engagement in "My Child's Asthma" an interactive web-based pediatric asthma management intervention. Int J Med Inform 2011;80(11):765–74.
18. El Mallakh P, Howard PB, Inman SM. Medical and psychiatric comorbidities in children and adolescents: a guide to issues and treatment approaches. Nurs Clin North Am 2010;45(4):541–54.
19. Peterson-Sweeny K. The relationship of household routines to morbidity outcomes in childhood asthma. J Pediatr Nurs 2009;14(1):59–69.
20. Crocker D, Kinyota S, Dumitru G, et al. Effectiveness of home based, multi-trigger multicomponent interventions with an environmental focus for reducing asthma morbidity; a community guide systematic review. Am J Prev Med 2011; 41(2 Suppl 1):S5–32.
21. Butz AM. Shared decision making in school age children with asthma. Pediatr Nurs 2007;33(2):111–6.
22. Mizan SS, Shendell DG, Rhoads GG. Absence extended absence, and repeat tardiness related to asthma status among elementary school children. J Asthma 2011;48(3):228–34.
23. Moonie S. The relationship between school absence, academic performance, and asthma status. J Sch Health 2008;78(3):140–8.
24. Bruzzese J, Evans D, Kattan M. School Based asthma programs. J Allergy Clin Immunol 2009;124:195–200.
25. Collins JE. Mental, emotional, and social problems among school children with asthma. J Asthma 2008;45(6):489–93.
26. Lipstein EA. School absenteeism, health status, and health care utilization among children with asthma: associations with parental chronic disease. Pediatrics 2009;123(1):360–6.
27. National Association of School Based Health Centers. Available at: http://www. nasbhc.org/site/c.ckLQKbOVLkK6E/b.7697107/apps/s/content.asp?ct=10884071. Accessed August 7, 2012.
28. Tai T, Bame S. Cost-benefit analysis of childhood asthma management through school based clinic programs. J Community Health 2011;36(2):253–60.

29. Putman-Casdorph H, Badzek L. Asthma and allergy medication self-administration by children in school: liability issues for the nurse. J Nurs Law 2011;14(1):32–6.
30. Allergy and Asthma Network Mothers of Asthmatics. Available at: http://www.aanma.org/advocacy/meds-at-school/. Accessed August 7, 2012.
31. Cicutto L. Supporting successful asthma management in schools: the role of the asthma care providers. J Allergy Clin Immunol 2009;124(2):390–3.
32. Chini L. Happy Air, a successful school based asthma educational and interventional program for primary school children. J Asthma 2011;48(4):419–26.
33. Bruzzese JM. Asthma knowledge and asthma management behavior in urban elementary school teachers. J Asthma 2010;47(2):185–91.
34. Okay with Asthma! Available at: www.okaywithasthma.org. Accessed August 7, 2012.
35. Wyatt RH, Hauenstein EJ. Pilot testing okay with asthma: an online asthma intervention for school-age children. J Sch Nurs 2008;24(3):145–50.
36. Jones SE, Wheeler LS, Smith AM, et al. Adherence to national Asthma Education and Prevention Program's "how asthma-friendly is your school?" recommendations. J Sch Nurs 2009;25(5):382–94.
37. Wilson K, Moonie S, Sterling D, et al. Examining the consulting physician model to enhance the school nurse role for children with asthma. J Sch Health 2009;79(1): 1–7.

Asthma Network of West Michigan

A Model of Home-based Case Management for Asthma

Karen L. Meyerson, MSN, RN, FNP-C, AE-C

KEYWORDS

- Asthma • Case management • Certified asthma educators • Reimbursement
- Asthma disparities

KEY POINTS

- This article presents an overview of the Asthma Network of West Michigan, the local asthma coalition serving West Michigan, and its intensive home-based case management model for individuals with uncontrolled asthma.
- The Asthma Network is believed to be the first grassroots asthma coalition in the nation to contract with health plans and obtain reimbursement for these services.
- The Asthma Network's program, using certified asthma educators and licensed masters-level social workers, has had a positive impact on health care use as well as cost savings, and its model has been replicated in other communities.

Asthma, the most prevalent chronic disease of children, is the leading cause of preventable pediatric hospitalizations in Michigan[1] and nationally is responsible for more school and daycare absenteeism than any other disease (more than 10 million days of school are missed each year because of asthma).[2] Unfortunately, as we have developed more effective treatments for asthma, we have not seen a corresponding decrease in asthma morbidity. According to Wasilevich and Lyon-Callo[3]:

> Asthma presents a significant burden to the residents of Michigan. Despite improvements in asthma management, preventable events (such as hospitalizations and death) still occur. Although there are many positive aspects to asthma management in Michigan, there are clear areas for improvement, as evidenced by disparities in asthma rates between racial groups and by income level. (p. 79)

Funding Sources: Spectrum Health, Saint Mary's Healthcare, First Steps Kent, Heart of West Michigan United Way, Priority Health, Amway.
Conflict of Interest: Speakers' Bureau – GlaxoSmithKline; Advisory Board – Ideomed, Inc.
Asthma Network of West Michigan, 359 South Division Avenue, Grand Rapids, MI 49503, USA
E-mail address: meyersok@trinity-health.org

Asthma cannot be cured, but it can be controlled. With appropriate chronic disease management, people with asthma can prevent asthma symptoms during the day and night and maintain normal activity levels. If asthma is adequately managed, individuals should not experience sleep disruption or miss days of school or work because of their asthma. They should also have minimal need for emergency department (ED) visits or hospitalizations owing to asthma. In fact, with proper asthma self-management, most ED visits, admissions, and asthma deaths are completely preventable.[4]

In reality, however, asthma imposes a significant and growing burden on society in terms of morbidity, quality of life, and health care costs, with a higher level of asthma burden associated with lower income and education levels.[5] Approximately 7 million children age 0–17 in the United States have asthma, with poor and minority children suffering a disproportionate burden of the disease.[2] Despite incredible advances in asthma care and the growth in asthma education programs and detailed asthma treatment guidelines, the asthma epidemic has hit our inner cities hardest, although there has been a substantial increase in asthma cases in suburban populations as well. Poverty, dire psychosocial problems, and poor medical care undoubtedly play a major role in the frequency and severity of asthma and are also important predicators for an asthma death.[6–8] Differences in the burden of asthma may also be related to social and economic status, access to health care, and exposure to environmental triggers.

Research shows that a targeted home-based asthma education intervention can be effective for improving health outcomes in children with asthma.[9,10] The National Institutes of Health acknowledges that the indoor environment is an important factor in the growing asthma problem.[4] According to the US Environmental Protection Agency,[11] the use of home visits to incorporate environmental risk factor management into traditional asthma management programs offers many benefits. A home visit provides an ideal setting to educate, review medication plans, and help families identify environmental factors in their homes that may contribute to the severity of asthma. The strategy of reducing exposures to environmental triggers is also consistent with and supports the national asthma guidelines.[4]

A MODEL OF CASE MANAGEMENT

The Asthma Network of West Michigan (ANWM), based in Grand Rapids, is the local asthma coalition that serves Western Michigan, and has been in existence for 18 years. It was formed in early 1994 in response to growing concern over pediatric asthma morbidity and mortality in Western Michigan. In 1996, to increase its community impact, the Asthma Network created a direct service arm for its coalition, using funding from local foundations and health care institutions and implemented home-based asthma case management services for school-age children who had uncontrolled asthma in Kent County.[12] In 1997, ANWM applied for and received 501(c)(3) nonprofit status. Since then, ANWM has expanded its reach to children younger than 5 years and to adults and now serves 3 Western Michigan counties. The Asthma Network's target population includes children and adolescents with uncontrolled asthma from low-income families who are covered by managed Medicaid (or may be uninsured), who miss many days of school, and have experienced hospitalizations or emergency room visits because of asthma.

These children are targeted specifically because of significant racial and ethnic disparities that exist for children with asthma, especially those living in poverty. Nationally, 12.2% of children with a family income less than 100% of the federal poverty level have asthma—compared with 9.9% of children with a family income up to 200% of the federal poverty level, and 8.2% of children with a family income greater than 200% of the federal poverty level.[13] In addition to disparities in the prevalence of asthma, there are significant racial and ethnic disparities in asthma outcomes (eg, measures of asthma control, exacerbation of symptoms, quality of life, health care use, and death).[13] Although asthma deaths are relatively rare, black children are 4 times more likely to die of asthma than white children nationwide,[13] compared with Michigan, where asthma deaths for black children occur at a rate 6 times that of white children.[14]

The mission of ANWM is to improve the health and quality of life of individuals with asthma, providing both educational and professional expertise. This directly relates to its 2 different, but complementary, interventions: (1) community outreach, which provides education about asthma (to more than 50,000 individuals since 1996) via regularly scheduled school, medical and allied professional conferences, using specially trained physicians, nurses, and respiratory therapists and (2) home-based asthma case management services for individuals with uncontrolled asthma (more than 4000 since 1996) through individual home visits in Kent, Ottawa, and Muskegon counties.

ANWM's model of education involves sending a certified asthma educator—a nurse (at the RN level) or respiratory therapist (at the RRT level)—into the homes of patients for up to a year to perform environmental assessments and to teach them (and their caregivers) about asthma pathophysiology, trigger identification and avoidance/reduction, medications, proper use of devices, and other self-management techniques. Spacers are given to all patients who do not have them. Asthma educator in-home visits typically are biweekly for 3 months to cover a set curriculum and then monthly thereafter for up to a year to reinforce earlier lessons and discuss or troubleshoot challenges. Patients generally graduate from ANWM, that is, no longer need its services because their asthma has sufficiently improved, by approximately 6–12 months.

In 2007, the National Asthma Education and Prevention Program Expert Panel Report 3 issued the first comprehensive update of the clinical practice guidelines for the diagnosis and management of asthma in a decade.[4] The guidelines emphasize the importance of asthma control and introduce new approaches for monitoring asthma. As a result, ANWM's clinical staff uses the Asthma Control Test—a standardized, validated questionnaire—to measure the level of asthma control at regular intervals (every 4 weeks). The guidelines also confirm the importance of teaching patients skills to self-monitor and manage asthma and to use a written asthma action plan, which should include instructions for daily treatment and ways to recognize and handle worsening asthma.[4] New recommendations encourage expanding educational opportunities to reach patients in a variety of settings, such as pharmacies, schools, community centers, and patients' homes, underscoring the hallmark of ANWM services: home-based asthma case management.

Asthma educators employed by the Asthma Network must be certified asthma educators (certification is achieved by passing the National Asthma Educator Certification Board examination) when hired or become certified within 1 year of employment. ANWM pays for the certification and recertification by examination every 7 years. Although asthma education is provided by the asthma educators or case managers, licensed masters-level social workers (LMSWs) provide psychosocial interventions for higher-risk families, assist parents with coping and parenting skills, and coordinate other services (housing, transportation, prescription coverage, and counseling referrals). ANWM's case management team arms parents with the tools and language essential to assess their child's daily condition. ANWM's in-home case management truly transforms whole families, as children are able to attend school, participate in sports, and learn to control their asthma. Addressing communication and psychosocial issues also strengthens the family. ANWM's in-home asthma case management services include coordinating the child's asthma action plan with a health care provider and providing asthma education or consultative services to the child's school or day care center.

ASTHMA ACTION PLANS

Asthma education and the use of written asthma action plans have been proven to reduce the burden of the disease when patients learn to manage asthma as a chronic, rather than episodic, condition.[4,15,16] Written asthma action plans provide a way to involve the patient directly in self-management. Reviewing the asthma action plan with the asthma educator is a perfect opportunity to identify if a patient is:

- Taking medications as prescribed
- Using correct inhaler/spacer device technique(s)
- Recognizing signs of worsening asthma and knowing which actions to take
- Keeping asthma under control

Asthma educators work with each child and his or her family and school and caregivers to reduce asthma triggers, identify ideal usage of medication and therapeutic devices (eg, inhalers), recognize the signs of an approaching attack, and help reduce the number and severity of the attacks. ANWM's case managers (including interpreters serving an ever-increasing Spanish-speaking caseload) also provide culturally sensitive home-based asthma education and case management services, eliminating language barriers and reviewing a written asthma action plan in their native language. They help the families communicate with their health care provider/medical home to achieve better control of their child's asthma through regular care conferences and phone calls with the health care provider/medical home staff.

PSYCHOSOCIAL SUPPORT

Although ANWM uses strategies predicated on the evidence-based Expert Panel Report 3 guidelines for asthma,[4] its interdisciplinary team delivers an innovative and effective program of in-home asthma education and case management. Key to its innovative approach is the use of LMSWs, whose services augment the clinical case management team. Although the case managers focus on specific asthma management and control issues, the LMSWs help families access additional resources to meet basic needs. ANWM's case-managed families typically have multiple stressors, ranging from environmental to financial to socio-legal; the use of the LMSWs to identify and assist with a family's problems leads to greater effectiveness in caring for the child's asthma as ANWM makes appropriate referrals or contacts to financial resources, mental health agencies, food banks, hospitals, and landlords, among others.

The Asthma Network LMSWs work intensively with the case-managed families, identifying areas of stress and financial need and assessing the mental health of both caregivers and children. These problems have been found to interfere with a caregiver's or patient's ability to adhere to treatment.[7] Through LMSW assessments, referrals, psychosocial interventions and follow-up, the strength and resilience of the family are supported to ensure successful management of asthma in a family-centered care environment.[12] With resources and support, families have a greater ability to focus on the proper management of asthma, and health outcomes improve.[17]

ASTHMA NETWORK OUTCOMES

Outcomes data are key indicators for measuring success for any asthma program. As noted by Williams and colleagues[18]:

ANWM measures many variables and shares the findings with financial decision makers. Although not previously published, ANWM outcomes data have been disseminated at numerous national and international medical conferences through poster presentations and lectures. The data support the benefits of the ANWM program in terms of fewer emergency room visits, hospitalizations, and overall costs for asthma care. (p. S12)

ANWM directly improves the health and well being of children and adults by providing in-home asthma education and case management to the underserved, uninsured, and underinsured. Data presented at national conferences over the last 18 years have shown significant reductions in the number of hospitalizations and days hospitalized for its case-managed children.[19] Case management data showed significant reductions in hospitalizations (from 41 to 13) and days hospitalized (from 114 to 25) in 3 successive, combined, 2-year, before-after cohorts (n = 45) through its case management program. These reductions were highly significant ($P<.0001$) when compared with a matched control group (n = 39) that did not receive ANWM's services.[20]

REIMBURSEMENT FOR ASTHMA EDUCATION

In 1996, focusing on school-aged children with moderate to severe asthma, 34 children completed the first-year pilot program and showed significant reductions in admissions and length of stay, a cost savings of $55,000 from 1 year to the next in facility charges (professional fees were not tracked).[12,21] After 2 years of the pilot program, Asthma Network leaders took their data to the largest payer in West Michigan (Priority Health), showing reductions in health care use and cost savings. The Asthma Network asked Priority Health to refer their most at-risk patients to ANWM for a trial of case management for 1 year, and then if the outcomes were compelling, they would enter into an agreement to begin reimbursing the Asthma Network for its services.[12] The 1-year demonstration was successful, and Priority Health entered into an agreement in 1999. Under this contract—the first such contract between a grassroots asthma coalition and a health plan in the nation—Priority Health agreed to reimburse ANWM at the standard Medicaid rate for a skilled nursing visit, revenue code 551, for both asthma educators (regardless of discipline) and LMSWs alike.

Since its agreement with Priority Health in 1999, the Asthma Network has contracted with 4 additional health plans who reimburse at the same standard rate (for a skilled nursing visit) and revenue code as Priority Health. Four of five of these payers are Medicaid plans, with one commercial partner. Most of the families served by the Asthma Network are Medicaid eligible (typically 300 to 400 families are served per year), with children as the primary patients.[12] Generally, referrals come from the county's patient-centered medical home program, the local children's hospital, physician practices, EDs, local clinics, school and public health nurses, and partner health plans. To provide services, the Asthma Network relies on payer reimbursement (covering one third of its budget) and grant funding (two thirds of its budget). These grant dollars come from local hospitals, foundations, and the United Way and support services to patients without insurance. There is a waiting list for uninsured or underinsured individuals needing services, but they will eventually be served, and no one referred for asthma case management in the ANWM service area is turned away.[12]

Before enrollment in the ANWM case management program, members must receive authorization. On average, health plans authorize from 6 to 18 home visits and often do so after an ED visit or hospitalization. Typically, health plan members targeted for the Asthma Network's services are those with uncontrolled asthma from low-income families. The health plans are able to track their return on investment because they have access to outcomes data. It is with this information that the health plans measure success and renew contracts.[12] The Asthma Network has since expanded its services to adults and children with uncontrolled asthma (mostly disadvantaged and low-income) in 3 counties. Expansion into one of the counties was requested by a payer because they had so many at-risk members with asthma residing in that county.

PATIENT-CENTERED MEDICAL HOME PILOT

In 2008 there was a new initiative in Grand Rapids—a patient-centered medical home pilot—funded by a community collaborative called *First Steps*. The pilot's focus was on increasing access to care and reducing unnecessary ED visits in children covered by Medicaid. First Steps, deciding to focus on asthma in particular, approached the Asthma Network to see if they would provide home-based case management and asthma education services for children with Priority Health Medicaid coverage. The partner health plan also incentivized some private pediatric practices to absorb more Medicaid patients and increased their Medicaid reimbursement rates accordingly. The pilot allowed ANWM staff unprecedented access into the medical homes (private practices and clinics alike) and allowed for the subsequent development of dashboards on provider and practice performance. The dashboards tracked not only use of services but also provision of flu shots, asthma action plans, asthma control test scores, 6-month asthma follow-up visits, and spirometry.[12] The pilot also allowed ANWM to incorporate community health workers into the case management team for the first time. Community health workers advocate for case-managed families and serve as peer educators, offering interpretation and translation services, providing culturally appropriate health education and information, and providing some direct services such as environmental assessments for patients with asthma and their families.

CASE MANAGEMENT REPLICATION AND RESULTS

Asthma Network leaders feel compelled to share ANWM's successes with other asthma programs throughout the country who wish to replicate its home-based asthma case management model. In Michigan, the Genesee County Asthma Network was providing a home-based asthma case management program similar to that of the Asthma Network's for 10 years but never received reimbursement for these services. Four years ago, at a payer summit, Asthma Network payers shared the benefits and return on investment they have realized with Genesee County payers, and Genesee County Asthma Coalition now contracts with 4 health plans. In Washtenaw County, a school-based program converted to a home-based case management model repli-cating that of the Asthma Network, as that model was preferred by the health plan who now reimburses the program. These 3 communities have since participated in the Michigan MATCH (Managing Asthma through Case Management in Homes) study—comparing outcomes from their respective case management models. These outcomes are currently being analyzed, but preliminary data show a 60% decrease in ED visits ($P<.5$) and 83% decrease in hospitalizations ($P<.5$) as well as a 42% increase in pediatric quality-of-life scores ($P<.5$) and 36% increase in caregiver quality-of-life scores ($P<.5$) among patients enrolled in the case management programs offered in these 3 communities (O'Brien M, Lyon-Callo SK, Vorce T, et al, unpublished data, 2012).

The Asthma Network has received national recognition for its innovative case management model. In 2006, ANWM was recognized for its efforts by the US Environmental Protection Agency (EPA) as a National Model Asthma Program (one of 6 in the nation) and in 2008, was awarded the National Environmental Leadership Award in Asthma Management by the US EPA. As a result, as an official mentor for the US EPA, leaders of the Asthma Network have guided other organizations throughout the country in their efforts to successfully organize asthma networks and develop similar case management programs and receive many requests each year for such assistance.

The national guidelines recognize that individuals who are receiving evidence-based medical care and education for asthma are able to avert asthma crises, including emergency room visits, hospitalizations, and asthma deaths, all of which are ultimately preventable.[4] Yet, this is not the case for every child with asthma because of asthma disparities, which have multiple, complex, and interrelated sources.[22] Strategies to reduce asthma disparities include the need for routine assessment of access to care issues, financial barriers to disease management, psychosocial stressors, family dysfunction, behavioral health issues, and health literacy, all of which are addressed through the Asthma Network's case management program. The Asthma Network's dual approach of education and intensive case management has provided a comprehensive care continuum for the management of asthma in West Michigan. Nationally recognized as a model asthma program, it has had a positive impact on health care use among children and adults with asthma. The ANWM is striving every day to bring asthma under control in its community. Individuals with asthma should expect nothing less.

REFERENCES

1. Olszewski J, Wisdom K. Healthy Michigan 2010: Michigan surgeon generals' health status report. Michigan Department of Community Health; 2010. Available at: http://www.michigan.gov/documents/Healthy_Michigan_2010_1_88117_7.pdf. Accessed January 11, 2013.
2. Akinbami LJ, Mooreman JE, Bailey C, et al. Trends in asthma prevalence, health care use, and mortality in the United States, 2001-2010. Centers for Disease Control and Prevention, National Center for Health Statistics; 2012. Available at: http://www.cdc.gov/nchs/data/databriefs/db94.pdf. Accessed October 10, 2012.
3. Wasilevich EA, Lyon-Callo S. Epidemiology of asthma in Michigan: 2004 surveillance report. Bureau of Epidemiology, Michigan Department of Community Health; 2004. Available at: http://www.michigan.gov/documents/MIAsthmaSurveillance_2004_96083_7.pdf. Accessed January 11, 2013.
4. National Institutes of Health. Clinical practice guidelines: expert panel report 3: guidelines for the diagnosis and management of asthma. Rockville (MD): US Dept of Health and Human Services, National Institutes of Health; 2007. NIH publication 07–4051.
5. Fuhlbrigge AL, Adams RJ, Guilbert TW, et al. The burden of asthma in the United States: level and distribution are dependent on interpretation of the national asthma education and prevention program guidelines. Am J Respir Crit Care Med 2002;166:1044–9.
6. Akinbami LJ, Schoendorf KC. Trends in childhood asthma: prevalence, health care utilization and mortality. Pediatrics 2002;110(2):315–22.
7. Elliott R. Poor adherence to anti-inflammatory medication in asthma: reasons, challenges, and strategies for improved disease management. Dis Manag Health Outcome 2006;14(4):223–33.

8. Ortega AN, Goodwin RD, McQuaid EL, et al. Parental mental health, childhood psychiatric disorders, and asthma attacks in island Puerto Rican youth. Ambul Pediatr 2004;4:308–15.
9. Kattan M, Stearns S, Crain E, et al. Cost effectiveness of a home-based environmental intervention for inner-city children with asthma. J Allergy Clin Immunol 2005;116(5):1058–63.
10. Krieger J, Takaro T, Allen C, et al. The Seattle-King County health homes project: a randomized, controlled trial of a community health worker intervention to decrease exposure to indoor asthma triggers. Environ Health Perspect 2005; 95(4):642–59.
11. United States Environmental Protection Agency (EPA). Implementing an asthma home visit program: 10 steps to help health plans get started. Office of Air and Radiation Indoor Environments Division (6609J); 2005. EPA 402-K-05-006. Available at: http://www.epa.gov/asthma/pdfs/implementing_an_asthma_home_visit_program.pdf. Accessed January 11, 2013.
12. Centers for Disease Control and Prevention (CDC). Asthma self-management and comprehensive home visits: approaches to enhancing reimbursement. in press.
13. Environmental Protection Agency (EPA). President's task force on environmental health risks and safety risks to children: coordinated federal action plan to reduce racial and ethnic asthma disparities 2012. Available at: http://www.epa.gov/childrenstaskforce/federal_asthma_disparities_action_plan.pdf. Accessed October 12, 2012.
14. Wasilevich EA, Lyon-Callo S, Dombkowski KJ. Disparities in Michigan's asthma burden. Lansing (MI): Bureau of Epidemiology, Michigan Department of Community Health; 2005.
15. Gibson PG, Powell H, Wilson A, et al. Self-management education and regular practitioner review for adults with asthma. Cochrane Database Syst Rev 2009.
16. Schatz M, Rachelefsky G, Krishnan JA. Follow-up after acute asthma episodes: what improves future outcomes? J Allergy Clin Immunol 2009;124:S35–42.
17. Mitchell DK, Adams SK, Murdock KK. Associations among risk factors, individual resources and indices of school-related asthma morbidity in urban, school-aged children: a pilot study. J Sch Health 2005;75(10):375–83.
18. Williams D, Portnoy J, Meyerson KL. Strategies for improving asthma outcomes: a case-based review of successes and pitfalls. J Manag Care Pharm 2010;16: S1–15.
19. Kirk GM, Crooks J, Vanlwaarden D, et al. Improvements in educational, behavioral and clinical outcomes in low-income children with moderate to severe asthma using an NAEPP-based educational program 1999. Abstract presented at American Academy of Allergy, Asthma and Immunology 55th Annual Meeting. Orlando Florida; 1999.
20. Kirk GM, Prangley J, Meyerson KL. Improved Clinical Outcomes Among Low-Income Children Enrolled in an Asthma Case Management Program 2001. Abstract presented at American Thoracic Society (ATS) International Conference 97th Annual Meeting. San Francisco; 2001.
21. Kirk GM, Fecht JA, Meyerson KL. Reduced hospital charges resulting from a pediatric asthma case management program 2000. Abstract presented at American Thoracic Society (ATS) International Conference 96th Annual Meeting. Toronto; 2000.
22. Canino G, Garro A, Alvarez M, et al. Factors associated with disparities in emergency department use among Latino children with asthma. Ann Allergy Asthma Immunol 2012;108(4):266–70.

Index

Note: Page numbers of article titles are in **boldface** type.

Nurs Clin N Am 48 (2013) 185–192
http://dx.doi.org/10.1016/S0029-6465(13)00023-6
0029-6465/13/$ – see front matter © 2013 Elsevier Inc. All rights reserved.
nursing.theclinics.com

Moving?

Make sure your subscription moves with you!

To notify us of your new address, find your **Clinics Account Number** (located on your mailing label above your name), and contact customer service at:

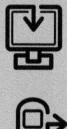

Email: journalscustomerservice-usa@elsevier.com

800-654-2452 (subscribers in the U.S. & Canada)
314-447-8871 (subscribers outside of the U.S. & Canada)

Fax number: 314-447-8029

Elsevier Health Sciences Division
Subscription Customer Service
3251 Riverport Lane
Maryland Heights, MO 63043

*To ensure uninterrupted delivery of your subscription, please notify us at least 4 weeks in advance of move.

Printed and bound by CPI Group (UK) Ltd, Croydon, CR0 4YY

03/10/2024

01040436-0013